THE Collagen Boost COOKBOOK

AF729769

THE Collagen Boost COOKBOOK

The secret ingredient to better hair, joints and skin in 60 delicious recipes

ELODIE COLOMBEL & SÉVERINE AUGÉ

@WIN.A.DIET

PHOTOGRAPHY BY FABRICE BESSE

hamlyn

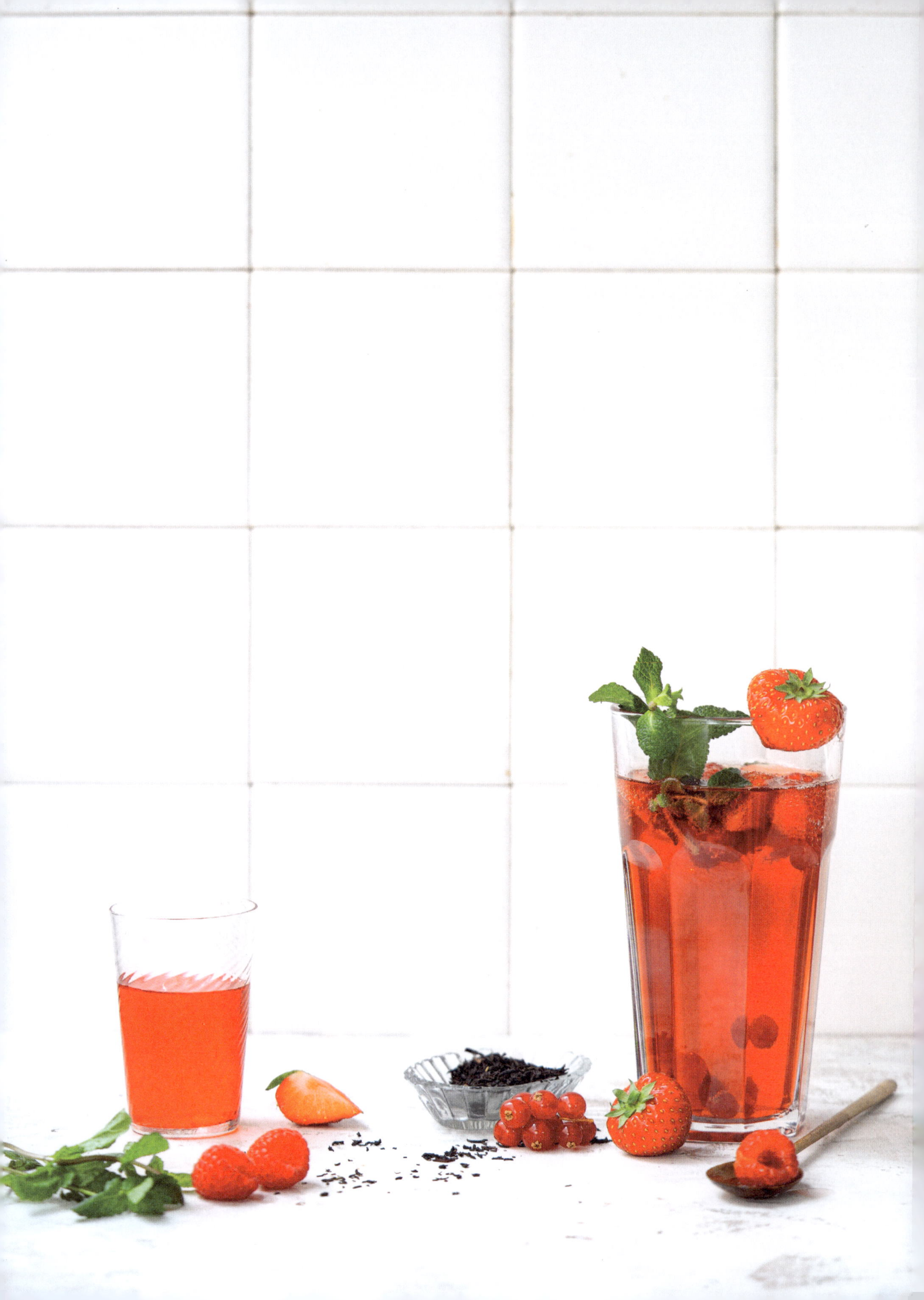

Contents

WHAT IS COLLAGEN?

Collagen is the most abundant protein in the human body, accounting for approximately 30% of the total protein mass. It is found in connective tissues (which help support other body tissues, providing nutrients as well as being involved in the body's immune defence mechanisms); it plays a crucial role in the structure and function of skin, bones, tendons, ligaments, joints, teeth and blood vessels; and it is what gives strength, elasticity and resilience to body tissues.

COLLAGEN: ROLE AND FUNCTION

Collagen acts as a type of **biological glue** that binds cells together. It also enables tissues to retain their shape and maintain cohesion.

- In the **skin**, it forms part of a valuable **support framework**, ensuring its elasticity, firmness and resistance to damage.
- In **joints**, it forms **cartilage,** which protects the bones from rubbing against each other and ensures mobility. It is also vital for the **structure of tendons and ligaments**, which connect muscles and bones and provide stability to the body during movement.
- It also provides **strength to blood vessels**, supporting vascular circulation.

COLLAGEN PRODUCTION REDUCES WITH AGE

After the age of about 25, our bodies start to produce less collagen, and this reduction speeds up over time. Once we hit 30 years old, **collagen synthesis** can drop by 1% a year. This progressive loss leads to visible and noticeable signs of ageing:

- **reduced skin elasticity** and a greater tendency to fine lines and wrinkles;
- **stiffer joints,** which predisposes them to wear and tear, sometimes making them painful;
- **reduced bone density**, leading to an increased risk of fractures and osteoporosis;
- **loss of skin volume and firmness**, particularly around the face and neck;
- **diminished regenerative capacity of tissues**, which slows down the healing process.

However, even if collagen production reduces with age, **it is possible to boost it by making adjustments to your diet**, using targeted external care and leading a healthy lifestyle.

In this book, we share recipes that will supplement your collagen naturally or help you boost collagen production.

HOW IS COLLAGEN SYNTHESIZED?

Collagen is made from special cells called fibroblasts, which are found in the skin and tissues. Collagen production involves several stages and follows quite a complex process.

STAGE 1 – THE SYNTHESIS OF AMINO ACIDS

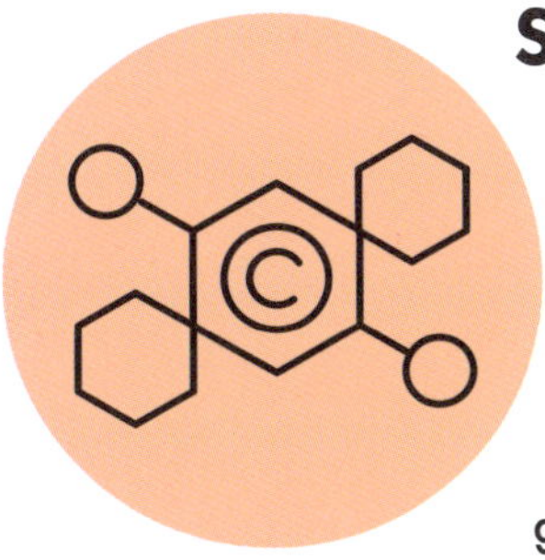

The first stage of collagen formation starts with the production of **essential amino acids: glycine, proline, lysine and hydroxylysine.** These amino acids are derived from **proteins** that we consume as part of our diet. To support **optimal synthesis,** it is essential to include protein sources with the **most comprehensive** amino acid profile possible in your diet.

STAGE 2 – THE VITAL ROLE OF VITAMIN C

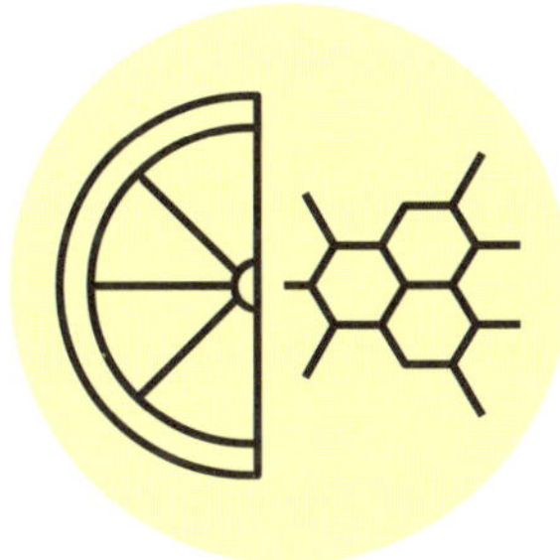

Vitamin C is essential for collagen formation, helping to convert the amino acids into collagen. It also helps to strengthen the collagen structurally, making it more robust and effective.

STAGE 3 – COLLAGEN SELF-ASSEMBLY

Once converted, the amino acids help to make procollagen, a preliminary form of collagen, inside the specialized skin cells. These molecules then assemble as **collagen fibres,** which migrate through the tissues to give them their essential properties such as **elasticity, firmness and cohesion.**

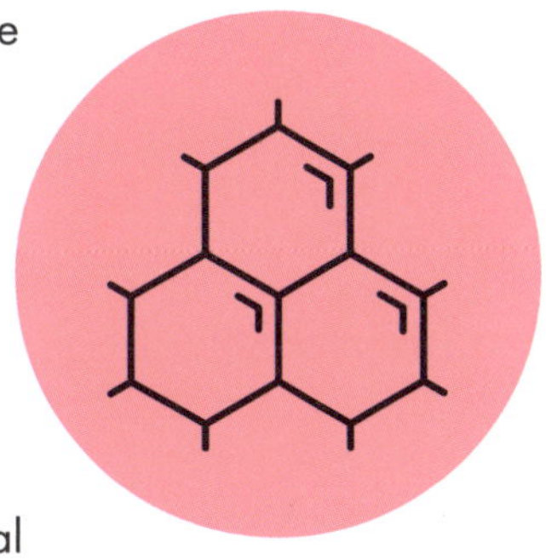

WHERE IS COLLAGEN FOUND?

Collagen can be found in various forms in our food. Some sources provide collagen, while others boost its natural synthesis. For each recipe in this book, a badge will indicate the purpose of the recipe – whether it provides supplementary collagen or boosts its production.

As a supplement

DIRECT SOURCES OF COLLAGEN

Foods rich in collagen are mainly found in animal proteins. It is the connective tissues of animals, such as skin, bones and cartilage, that are particularly rich in collagen. By consuming them, you are providing your body with a direct source of collagen.

1 **Bone broth (chicken, beef or fish)**, made using chicken, beef or fish bones, is one of the best sources of collagen.

2 **Fish and chicken skin** are very rich in marine and avian collagen. Chicken and duck skin, as well as skin from fish such as salmon, are particularly rich in collagen.

3 **Gelatine, derived from skin and bone,** is a hydrolysed form of collagen. This is a transformed collagen that is easily assimilated by the body.

4 **Pigs' feet, beef cheeks, tendons and marrow bones**, the parts of animals that are often ignored, have the highest concentrations of collagen.

5 **Beef and chicken cartilage** are rich in Type II collagen, ideal for joints.

To **boost** production

COLLAGEN BOOSTERS

Our bodies need certain foods and nutrients to optimize collagen production.

Foods and nutrients that boost collagen synthesis:

1

Foods rich in vitamin C (an essential cofactor in collagen synthesis). They include:

- citrus fruit (oranges, lemons, grapefruit);
- kiwifruit;
- berries (blackcurrants, strawberries, blueberries, goji berries, etc.);
- red and yellow peppers;
- parsley, coriander, chives;
- broccoli, Brussels sprouts, kale.

2

Zinc and copper.
Zinc activates the enzymes necessary for collagen production, and copper plays a part in the formation of cross-links between the collagen fibres. They can be found in:

- oysters, seafood, calves' liver;
- pumpkin seeds, cashew nuts, sesame seeds;
- raw cacao and dark chocolate (85% cocoa solids).

3

Amino acids essential for collagen production. They can be found in:

- egg white;
- lean meat and fish;
- legumes (lentils, chickpeas, kidney beans etc.);
- seeds and nuts.

4

Silica is a mineral that stabilizes collagen. It can be found in:

- garlic, onion, shallots;
- eggs;
- cabbage, black radish, asparagus.

5

Omega-3 fatty acids protect and regenerate collagen. They reduce inflammation by protecting the collagen fibres from damage caused by oxidative stress. They can be found in:

- oily fish;
- flaxseeds, hemp seeds and camelina seeds;
- nuts and chia seeds;
- chicken and eggs.

6

Antioxidants and polyphenols combat collagen breakdown. They reduce inflammation and neutralize free radicals, which can damage collagen and accelerate ageing. They can be found in:

- green tea and matcha;
- tomatoes;
- pomegranate.

OUTSIDE OF YOUR DIET: TAKING CARE OF YOUR BODY

Food is just one element that helps boost collagen levels. It is just as important to take care of your body to maintain collagen levels overall.

- **Stay hydrated:** Collagen needs water to remain flexible and elastic. Adequate hydration is therefore essential for collagen preservation.

- **Sleep well:** Collagen regenerates during sleep, particularly during the deep sleep phases.

- **Moderate excercise:** Physical activity stimulates collagen production, especially for tendons and ligaments.

- **Manage stress:** Oxidative stress, caused by excessive stress or an unbalanced diet, can speed up collagen depletion.

- **Herbal infusions:** Some plants, such as nettle, horsetail or camomile, are renowned for their ability to stimulate collagen production.

- **Facial massage:** Performing stimulating massage on the skin improves blood circulation and helps with collagen production.

- **Steam baths:** To stimulate the absorption of nutrients through the skin and clean the pores, a steam bath made from herbs that are rich in silica is recommended.

- **Oils:** Oils rich in essential fatty acids and antioxidants, such as musk rose oil or grape seed oil, will nourish the skin and stimulate collagen production. They can be applied locally or be incorporated into your skin care regime.

Food supplements: Essential micronutrients (Omega-3, copper, zinc) will optimize collagen synthesis.

Various external factors will speed up collagen depletion.

- **Unbalanced diet:** Excessive sugar intake speeds up glycation and the depletion of collagen fibres.

- **Sun exposure:** It is recommended to use appropriate sunscreen to avoid damage caused by UV light, which also accelerates collagen depletion.

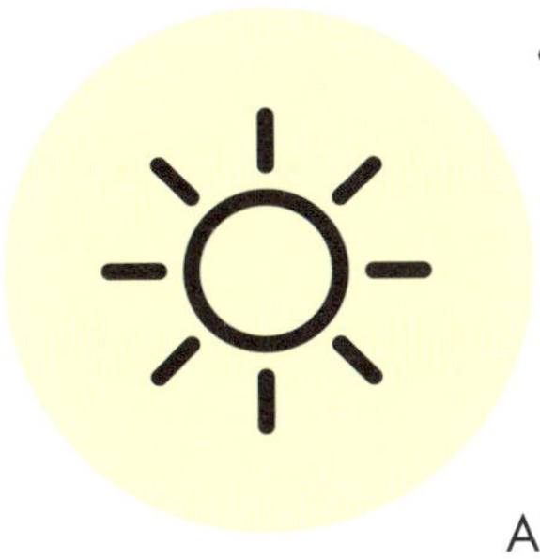

- **Smoking:** This should be avoided, as it can affect collagen production and speed up skin ageing.

- **Alcohol consumption:** Alcohol intake should be limited as it can also affect collagen production and speed up skin ageing.

- **Chronic stress:** This leads to the excessive production of cortisol, a hormone that can adversely affect collagen fibres. To reduce its impact, meditation, deep breathing or yoga can help to regulate cortisol, and therefore protect collagen.

- **Lack of sleep :** Restorative sleep (about 7–8 hours per night) is crucial for collagen rejuvenation.

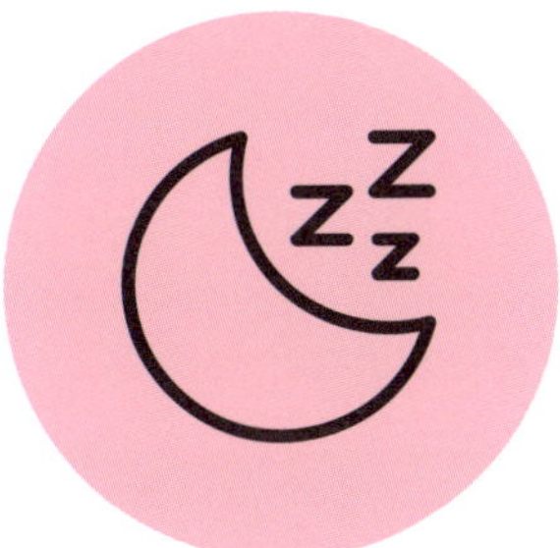

COLLAGEN SUPPLEMENTS: HOW TO CHOOSE THE RIGHT OFF-THE-SHELF PRODUCT

1

Collagen Types: I, II, III

- **Marine collagen** is more easily assimilated and is rich in Type I (for skin, hair and nails).
- **Bovine collagen** contains Types I and III (for skin and connective tissue).

2

Peptide size, molecular weight, daltons

A good collagen is hydrolysed (broken into small pieces) for better absorption. A molecular weight of between 2,000 and 5,000 daltons (2kDa and 5kDa) is most easily absorbed. The lower the weight, the better it can be assimilated.

3

The presence of vitamin C

Vitamin C is essential to stimulate collagen synthesis. Check that it has been added to your chosen collagen supplement.

4

Other active benefits (extras)

- **Hyaluronic acid:** hydrates the skin and boosts the collagen effect.
- **Zinc and silica:** support tissue regeneration.
- **Glycine and proline:** crucial amino acids for collagen production.

5

A clean and effective formulation

Choose a collagen without unnecessary additives or added sugar, preferably derived from a sustainable and traceable source.

COOKING METHODS FOR OPTIMAL COLLAGEN PRESERVATION

Collagen is a protein that is sensitive to heat and certain cooking methods. It is therefore essential to use gentle and slow cooking methods to preserve its structure and benefits. Here are the most suitable.

SLOW COOKING AT LOW TEMPERATURES

Long, slow cooks, such as stews, broths or ragùs, are ideal to extract collagen from the connective tissues of animals, particularly from bones and cartilage. They allow the collagen fibres to slowly dissolve in the water, or transform into gelatine, a form that is easily assimilated by the body. To make bone broth, it is recommended to cook the ingredients at a low temperature (around 80–90°C/176–194°F) for several hours, ideally 12–24 hours. This process extracts collagen efficiently without degrading it.

STEAM COOKING

This is a gentle cooking method because it preserves most of the nutrients, including collagen. By allowing the heat to gently circulate around the food, steaming preserves the texture and the bioactive properties of collagen, without any loss of liquid or nutrients. This is particularly true for oily fish, the skin of which is an excellent source of marine collagen.

PRESSURE COOKING

The pressure cooker is an excellent way to cook bone broths and collagen-rich meat dishes while considerably reducing cooking times. Thanks to the pressure, this method enables the rapid extraction of collagen from bones and tissues while preserving its quality and benefits. It is a fast and efficient option.

GENTLE OVEN COOKING

For some foods, such as chicken or fish, gentle oven cooking at low temperatures (around 150–160°C/300–325°F/Gas Mark 2–3) helps preserve skin and connective tissues without rendering them too dry or rubbery. It is recommended when cooking meat to keep the skin on and the collagen-rich parts intact.

Avoid

COOKING AT HIGH TEMPERATURES

Cooking at high temperatures, such as grilling, frying or sautéing, is to be avoided if you want to preserve collagen structure. The heat leads to a rapid degradation of the collagen fibres and significant losses of nutrients. Moreover, the high temperature can promote the formation of harmful compounds that affect the benefits of collagen and are detrimental to health.

Tips

Stock can be stored in the refrigerator for up to a week.

For a quick soup, remove any bay leaves or onion skins, then blitz the cooked vegetables with some of the stock.

You can buy fish stock from your fishmonger, kombu (edible seaweed) from a Japanese delicatessen or online, and fresh nettles from some greengrocers.

To remove the fat, allow the stock to cool completely before skimming off the layer of fat that forms on the surface.

Divide stock into small portions and store in an ice-cube tray in the freezer. This makes it easier to use in dishes for just one or two people, and it can be stored for longer! It can be stored frozen for up to six months.

Set aside the meat and shred the flesh to use in other recipes.

Broths, Stocks and Drinks

Chicken Stock

MAKES **4 LITRES (7 PINTS)**
PREPARATION TIME: **10 MINUTES** • COOKING TIME: **3½ HOURS**

- 1 bulb of garlic
- 3 carrots
- 2 celery sticks
- 2 onions
- 2 chicken carcasses (or 3 skin-on, bone-in chicken thighs)
- olive oil, for brushing
- 2 bay leaves
- 3 thyme sprigs
- 1 teaspoon peppercorns
- 5 litres (8¾ pints) water
- 20 g (¾ oz) dried mushrooms (porcini, morels, black mushrooms, etc.)

1. Preheat the oven to 200°C (400°F), Gas Mark 6.
2. Slice the garlic bulb in half, horizontally. Clean the vegetables, trim the ends off and chop into large pieces without peeling.
3. Place the chicken carcasses (or thighs) on a baking sheet or tray with the garlic halves, carrot, celery and onion pieces. Brush with olive oil and bake in the oven for 20 minutes.
4. Meanwhile, preheat the grill to hot, or 230°C (450°F).
5. Remove the chicken and vegetables from the oven, muddle the pieces around, then place under the grill for 5 minutes.
6. Transfer everything to a large casserole dish. Add the herbs, peppercorns and water before adding the dried mushrooms. Bring to the boil, then cover and cook at a gentle simmer for about 3 hours over a medium heat.
7. Once cooked, strain the stock.

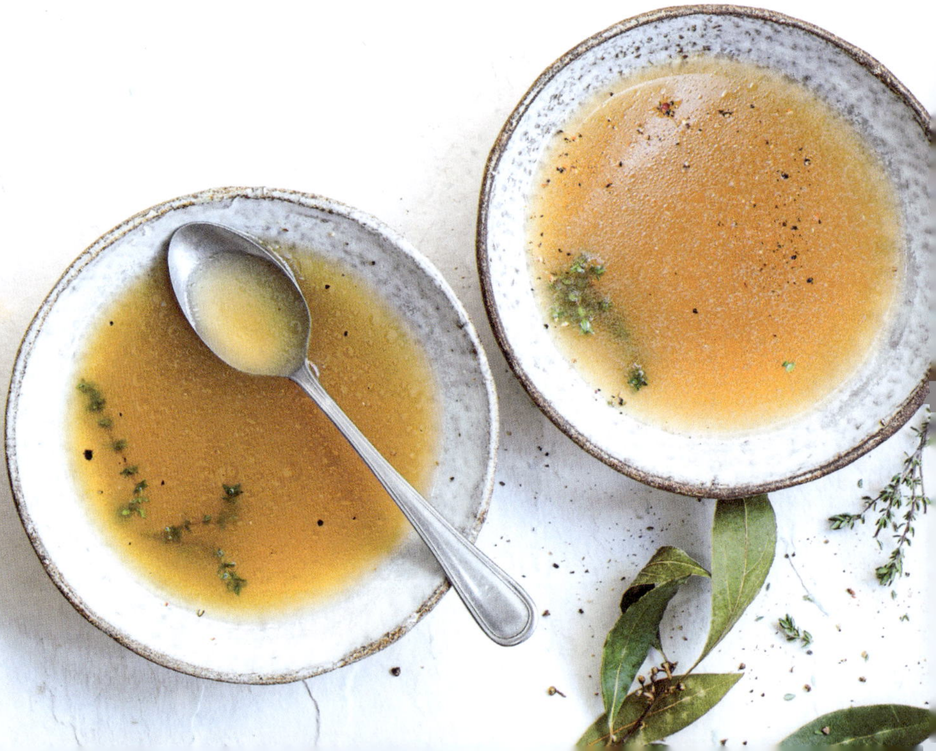

As a supplement

To boost production

'Pot-au-Feu' Broth

MAKES **2 LITRES (3½ PINTS)**
PREPARATION TIME: **10 MINUTES** • COOKING TIME: **4¼ HOURS**

- 1 tablespoon oil
- 1 onion, peeled and halved
- 1 kg (2 lb) beef (neck, chuck or oxtail), cut into pieces
- 3 litres (5½ pints) water
- 300 g (10 oz) veal or beef bones (optional)
- 4 carrots, peeled and cut into chunks
- 1 leek top (green part), washed and cut into chunks
- 8 cloves
- 1 bouquet garni
- 1 teaspoon coarse salt

1. Heat the oil in a casserole dish. When hot, add the onion halves, cut-sides down, and cook for about 5 minutes without moving until they are charred.
2. Meanwhile, place the meat in a separate large saucepan, cover with water and bring to the boil. Cook for 5 minutes (a grey foam with all the impurities will form on the surface).
3. Drain the meat, throw away the water and rinse the meat well.
4. Place the meat into the casserole dish with the onion halves and pour in the measured water. Add the remaining ingredients. Bring to the boil, then cover and cook at a gentle simmer for at least 4 hours over a medium heat.
5. Once cooked, strain the stock.

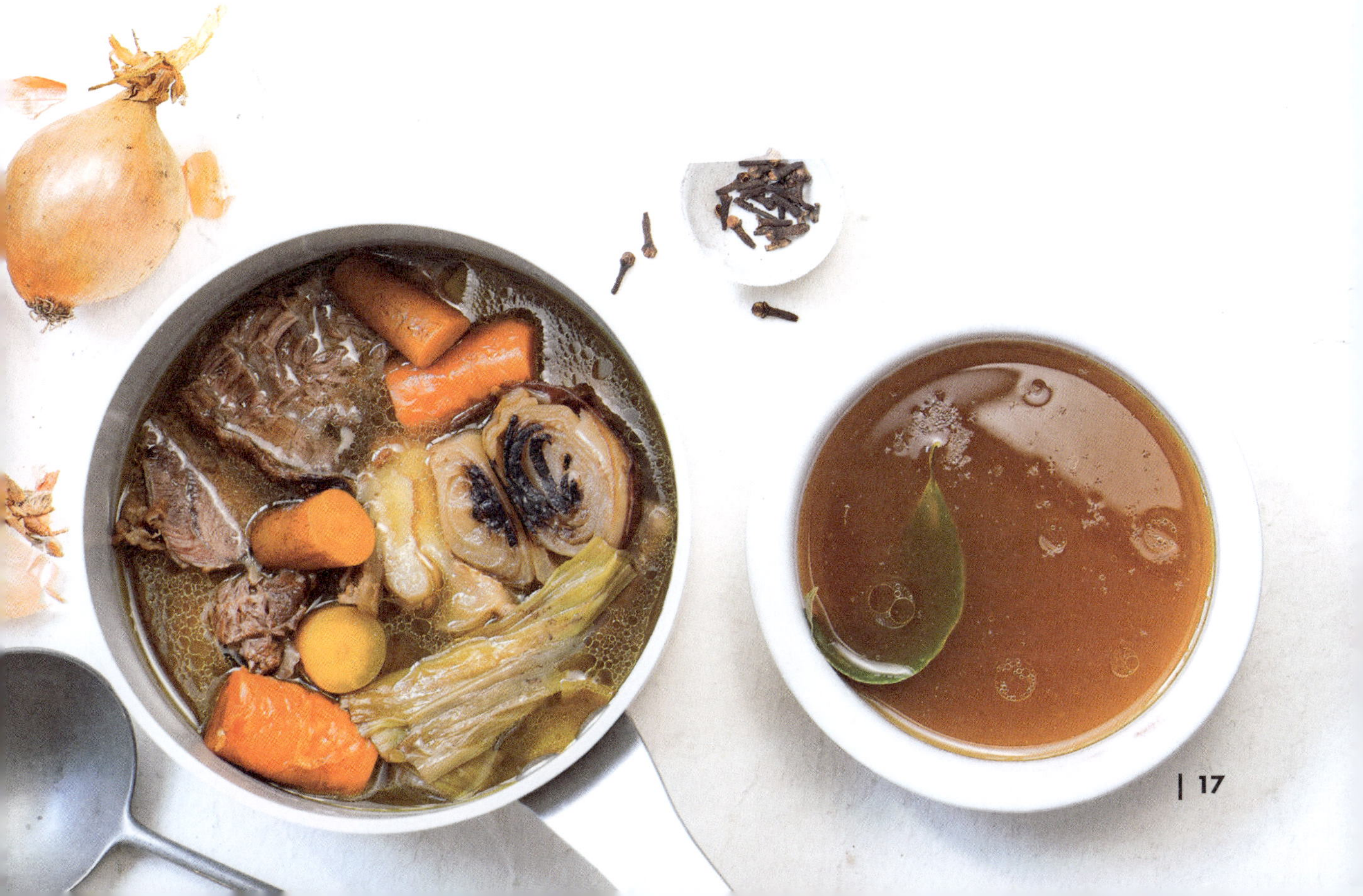

Phô Broth

As a supplement

MAKES **2 LITRES (3½ PINTS)**
PREPARATION TIME: **10 MINUTES** • COOKING TIME: **3¼–4¾ HOURS**

- 2 onions
- 30 g (1¼ oz) fresh root ginger
- splash of oil
- 300 g (10 oz) boneless beef chuck
- 500 g (1 lb) blade steak
- 500 g (1 lb) oxtail, cut into pieces (ask your butcher)
- 3 litres (5½ pints) water
- 4 garlic cloves, peeled and crushed
- 3 star anise
- 3 green cardamom pods, crushed with a pestle and mortar
- 4 cloves, crushed with a pestle and mortar
- 1 tablespoon coriander seeds
- 1 cinnamon stick
- 1 teaspoon coarse salt
- 2 tablespoons brown sugar
- 7 tablespoons nuoc-mâm (Vietnamese dipping sauce)

1. Rinse the onions and ginger without peeling, then halve them. Heat a splash of oil in a large casserole dish and char the ginger and onion halves, cut-sides down, until they start to blacken.
2. Meanwhile, place the meat in a separate large saucepan, cover with water and bring to the boil for 5 minutes (a grey foam with all the impurities will form on the surface).
3. Drain the meat, throw away the water and rinse the meat well.
4. Place the meat in the casserole dish with the charred ginger and onions and add the measured water. Add the garlic, spices, salt, brown sugar and nuoc-mâm. Bring to the boil, then cover and cook at a gentle simmer for 3–4½ hours over a medium heat.
5. Once cooked, strain the stock. Reserve the cooked meat for another recipe.

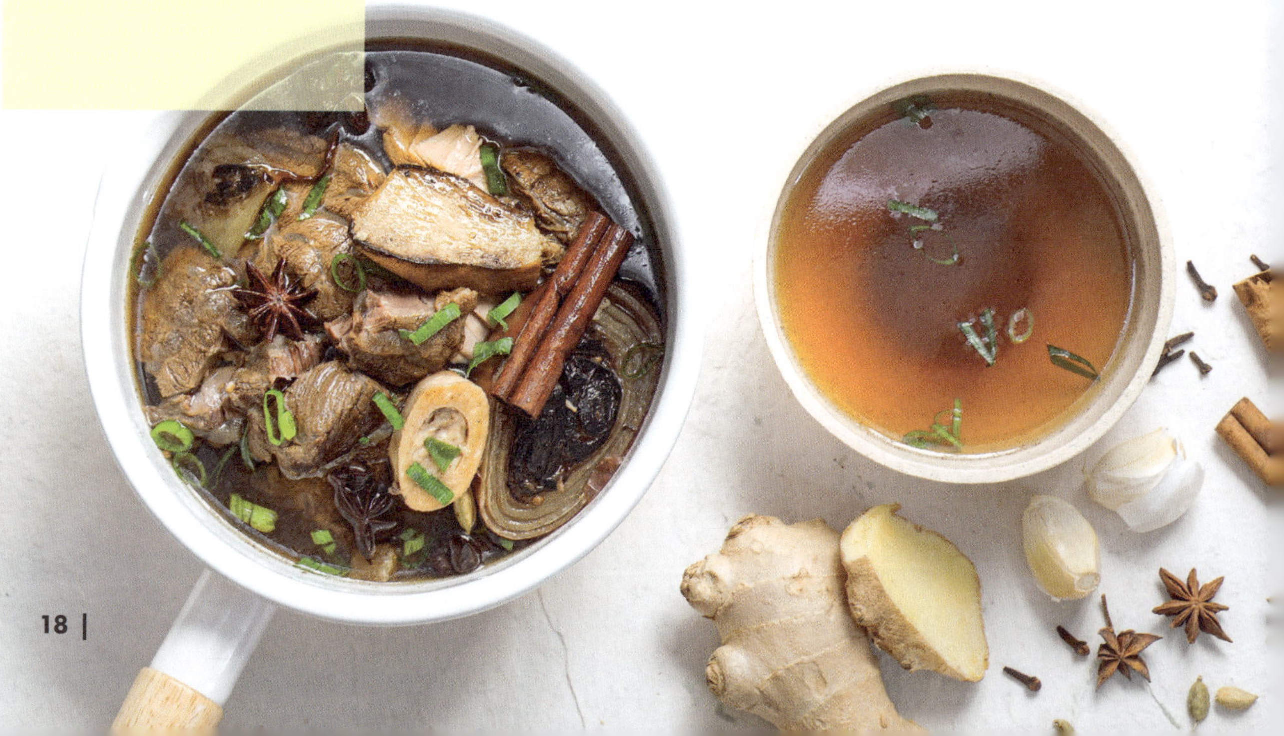

As a supplement

Pork Stock

MAKES **2 LITRES (3½ PINTS)**
PREPARATION TIME: **10 MINUTES** • COOKING TIME: **3¼ HOURS**

- 1 bone-in, rind-on ham hock (about 1.3 kg/2½ lb), cut into large pieces
- splash of oil
- 1 bulb of garlic, halved widthways
- 1 carrot, peeled and cut into large pieces
- 2 leeks, halved lengthways, thoroughly washed and cut into large pieces
- 1 rosemary sprig
- 3 thyme sprigs
- 1 bay leaf
- 1 teaspoon peppercorns, crushed
- 1 teaspoon coarse salt
- 3 litres (5½ pints) water

1. Place the meat in a large saucepan, cover with water and bring to the boil for 5 minutes (a grey foam with all the impurities will form on the surface).
2. Drain the meat, throw away the water and rinse the meat well.
3. Wash out the saucepan, then add a splash of oil and heat. When hot, add the garlic, cut-sides down, and quickly brown, then add the vegetables, herbs, peppercorns and salt. Place the pieces of meat on top, then add the measured water. Bring to the boil, then cover and cook at a gentle simmer for about 3 hours over a medium heat.
4. Once cooked, strain the stock. Shred the meat and reserve for another recipe.

Tip

If you prefer, you can use pork shoulder blade and shoulder instead of the ham hock.

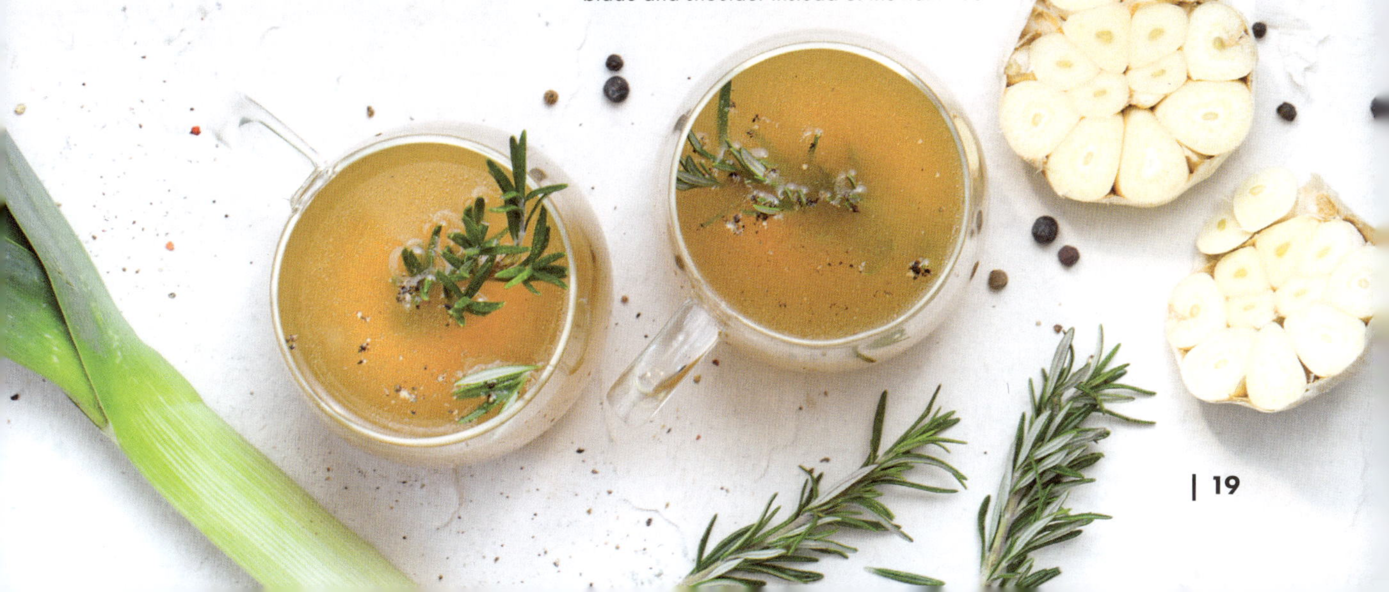

Fish Stock

MAKES **2 LITRES (3½ PINTS)**
PREPARATION TIME: **10 MINUTES** • COOKING TIME: **2 HOURS**
RESTING TIME: **MINIMUM 1½ HOURS**

As a **supplement**

To **boost** production

- 1.5 kg (3 lb) fish bones
- 2 carrots
- 2 shallots
- 1 leek (white part only)
- 2 celery sticks
- 3 litres (5½ pints) water
- 2 bay leaves
- 3 thyme sprigs
- 1 teaspoon juniper berries, crushed

1. The evening before (or at least 1½ hours beforehand), place the fish bones in a large bowl of cold water to soak. Replace the water once or twice during this period.
2. Rinse the vegetables and scrub well (do not peel the carrots and shallots) and trim the ends off. To clean the leek properly, cut it in half lengthways before rinsing. Cut all the vegetables into large pieces.
3. Place the drained bones in a large casserole dish with the vegetables. Add the measured water, then the herbs and juniper berries, and bring to the boil. Cover and cook at a gentle simmer for about 2 hours over a medium heat.
4. Once cooked, strain the stock.

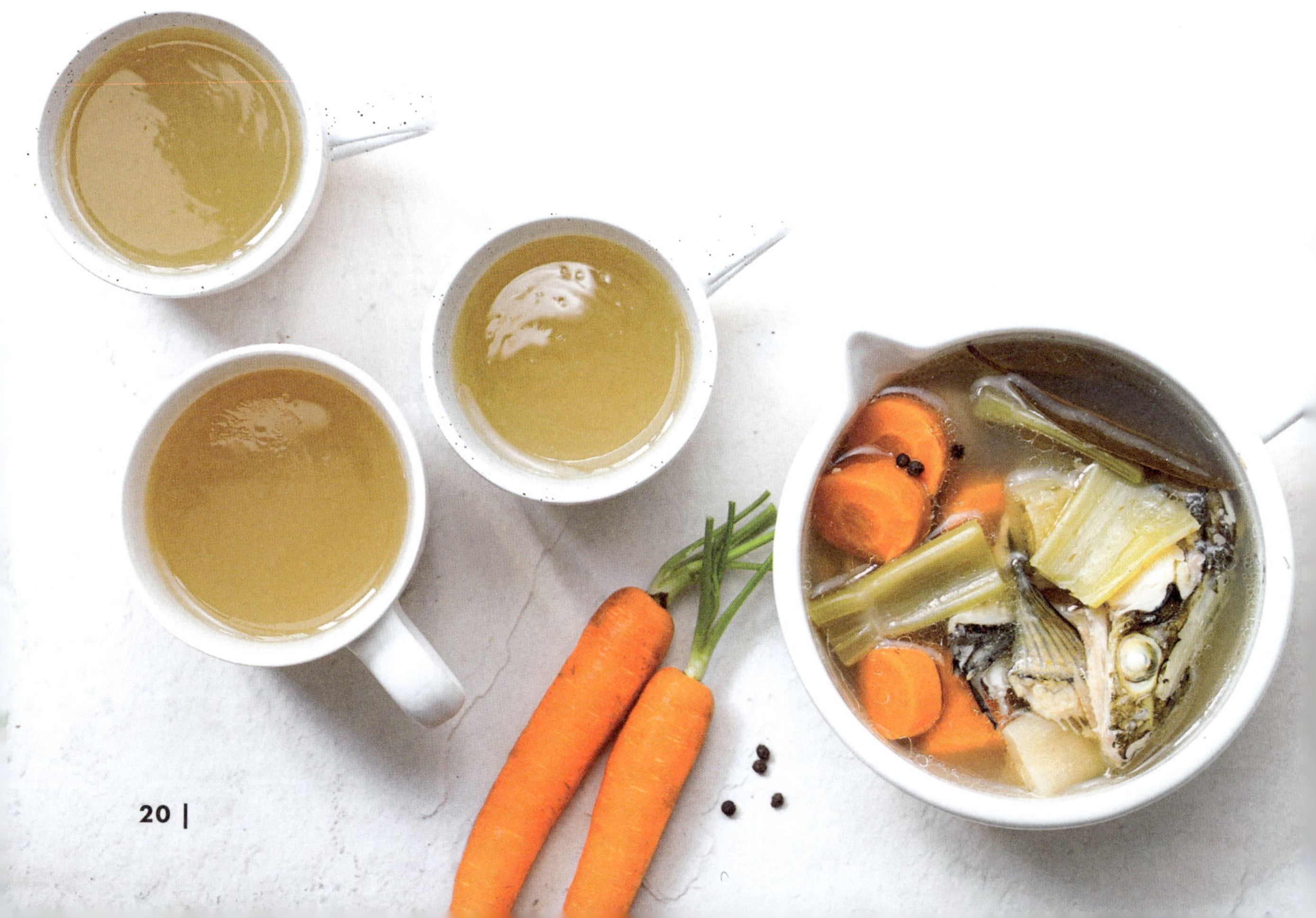

As a supplement

To boost production

Thai-style Prawn Broth

MAKES **2 LITRES (3½ PINTS)**
PREPARATION TIME: **10 MINUTES** • COOKING TIME: **2¼ HOURS**
RESTING TIME: **MINIMUM 1½ HOURS**

600 g (1 lb 4 oz) fish bones
1 tablespoon oil
4 spring onions, sliced
5 cm (2 inches) fresh root ginger (or galangal), sliced
about 20 raw king prawn shells
1 lemongrass stalk, lightly crushed
1 carrot, trimmed and cut into large pieces
2 celery sticks, trimmed and cut into large pieces
3 litres (5½ pints) water
6 dried lime leaves (optional)

1. The evening before (or at least 1½ hours beforehand), place the fish bones in a large bowl of cold water to soak. Replace the water once or twice during this period.
2. Heat the oil in a large saucepan until hot. Add the spring onions and ginger and sauté for 2 minutes, then add the drained fish bones and prawn shells. Cook for a further 5 minutes.
3. Add the crushed lemongrass, then add the carrot and celery chunks to the saucepan.
4. Pour in the measured water, add the dried lime leaves (if using) and bring to the boil. Cover and cook at a gentle simmer for about 2 hours over a medium heat.
5. Once cooked, strain the stock.

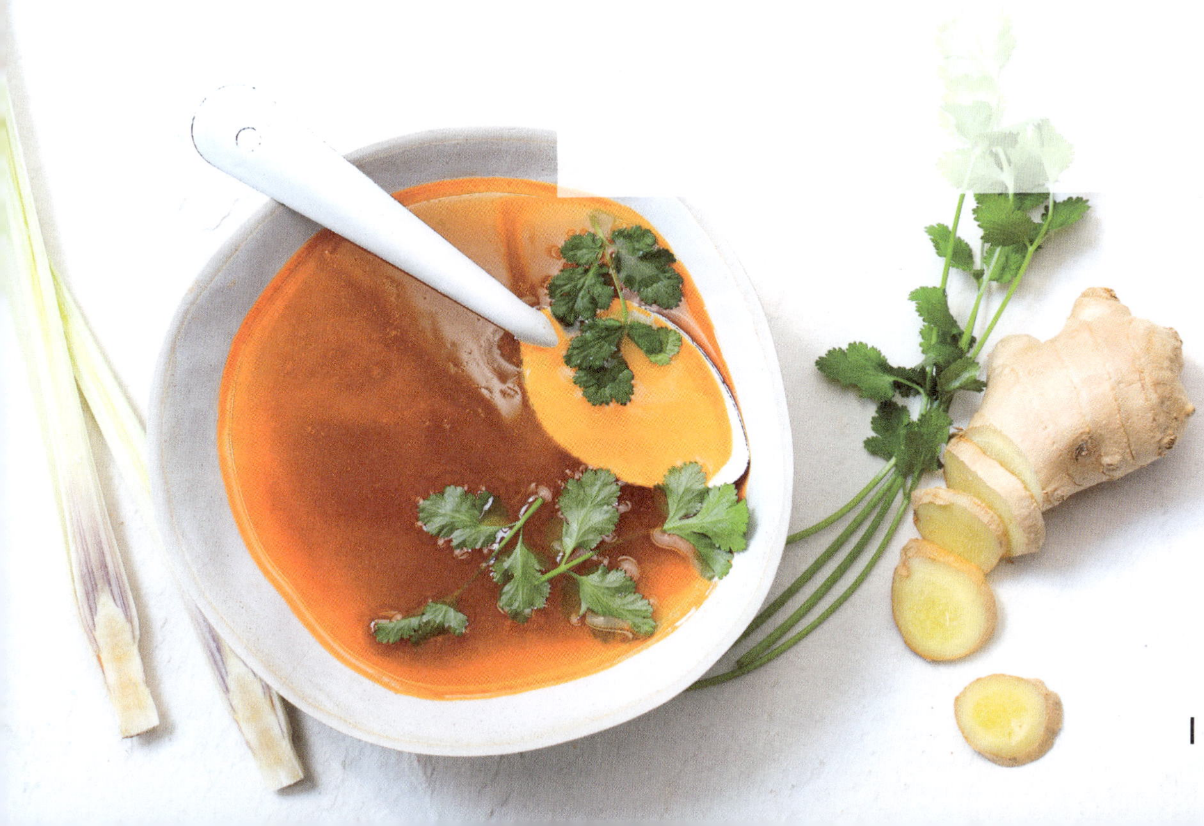

Dashi

To boost production

MAKES **2 LITRES (3½ PINTS)**
PREPARATION TIME: **5 MINUTES** • COOKING TIME: **10 MINUTES**
RESTING TIME: **35 MINUTES (FISH DASHI)–2¼ HOURS (VEGETARIAN DASHI)**

15 g (½ oz) kombu (edible seaweed)
2 litres (3½ pints) water
25 g (1 oz) katsuobushi (for fish dashi) or 4 shiitake mushrooms (for vegetarian dashi)

1. Quickly rinse the kombu and cut several notches along the edge with scissors (this improves the flavour infusion).
2. Place the kombu in a small saucepan with the measured water. Heat until small bubbles start to form in the water. Do not let it boil. Turn off the heat and leave to infuse for 15 minutes.
3. Remove the seaweed and reheat (without bringing to the boil), then add the katsuobushi (or shiitake mushrooms).
4. Turn off the heat and leave to infuse for 20 minutes for the katsuobushi version, or 2 hours for the shiitake version.
5. Strain and store for up to 6 days in an airtight container in the refrigerator.

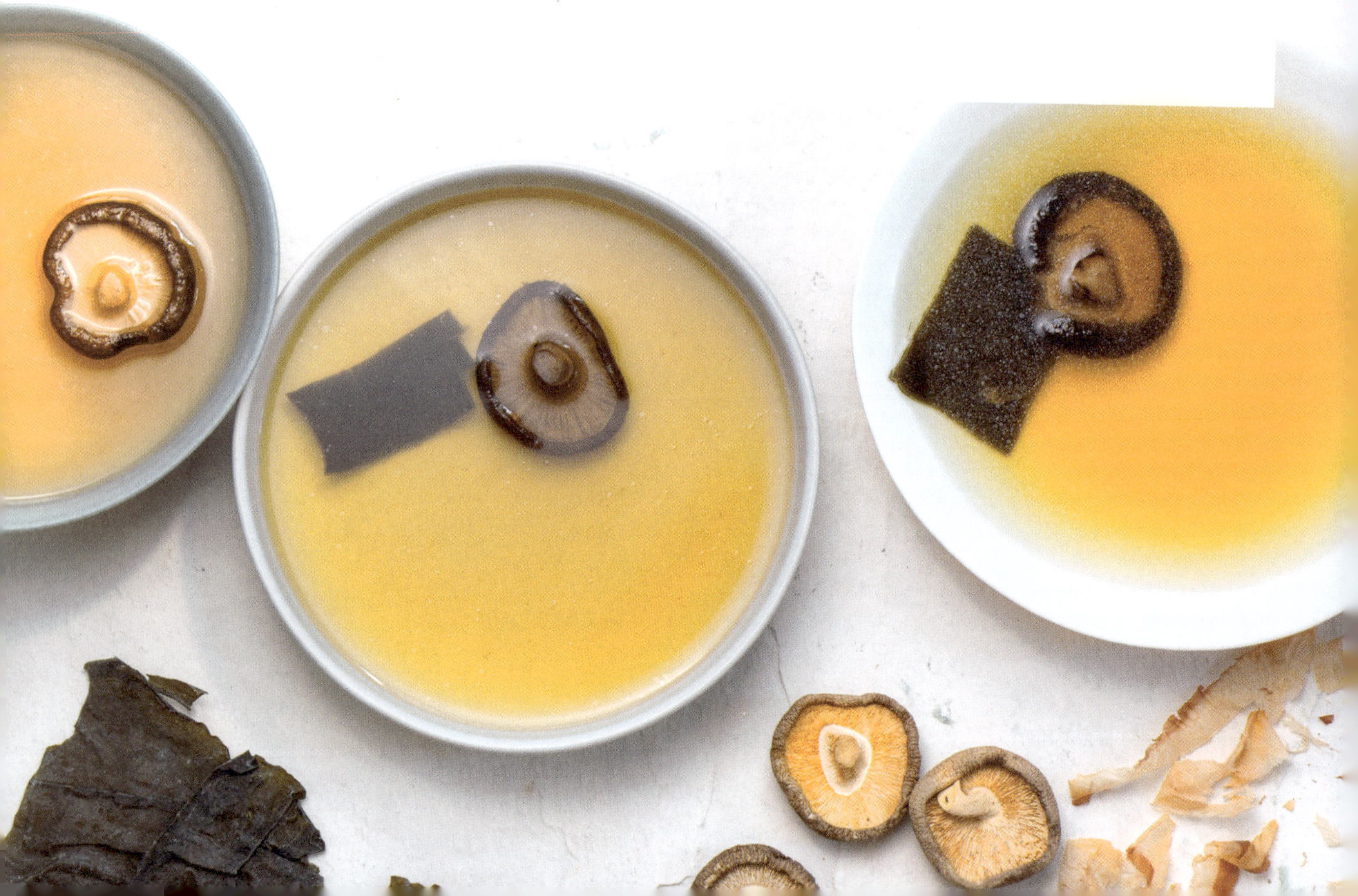

Vegetable Stock

To **boost** production

MAKES **2 LITRES (3½ PINTS)**
PREPARATION TIME: **10 MINUTES** • COOKING TIME: **1½ HOURS**

- 2 carrots
- 1 onion
- 2 celery sticks
- 1 leek
- 3 litres (5½ pints) water
- 1 teaspoon coarse salt
- 2 bay leaves
- 1 handful dried mushrooms (porcini or mixed)

1. Rinse and scrub the vegetables well (do not peel the carrots or onion). To clean the leek properly, cut it in half lengthways before thoroughly washing. Trim the vegetables and cut into large pieces.
2. Place all the vegetables into a casserole dish and pour in the measured water.
3. Add the salt, bay leaves and dried mushrooms and bring to the boil. Cover and cook at a gentle simmer for at least 1½ hours over a medium heat.
4. Strain the stock and store in the refrigerator for up to 7 days.

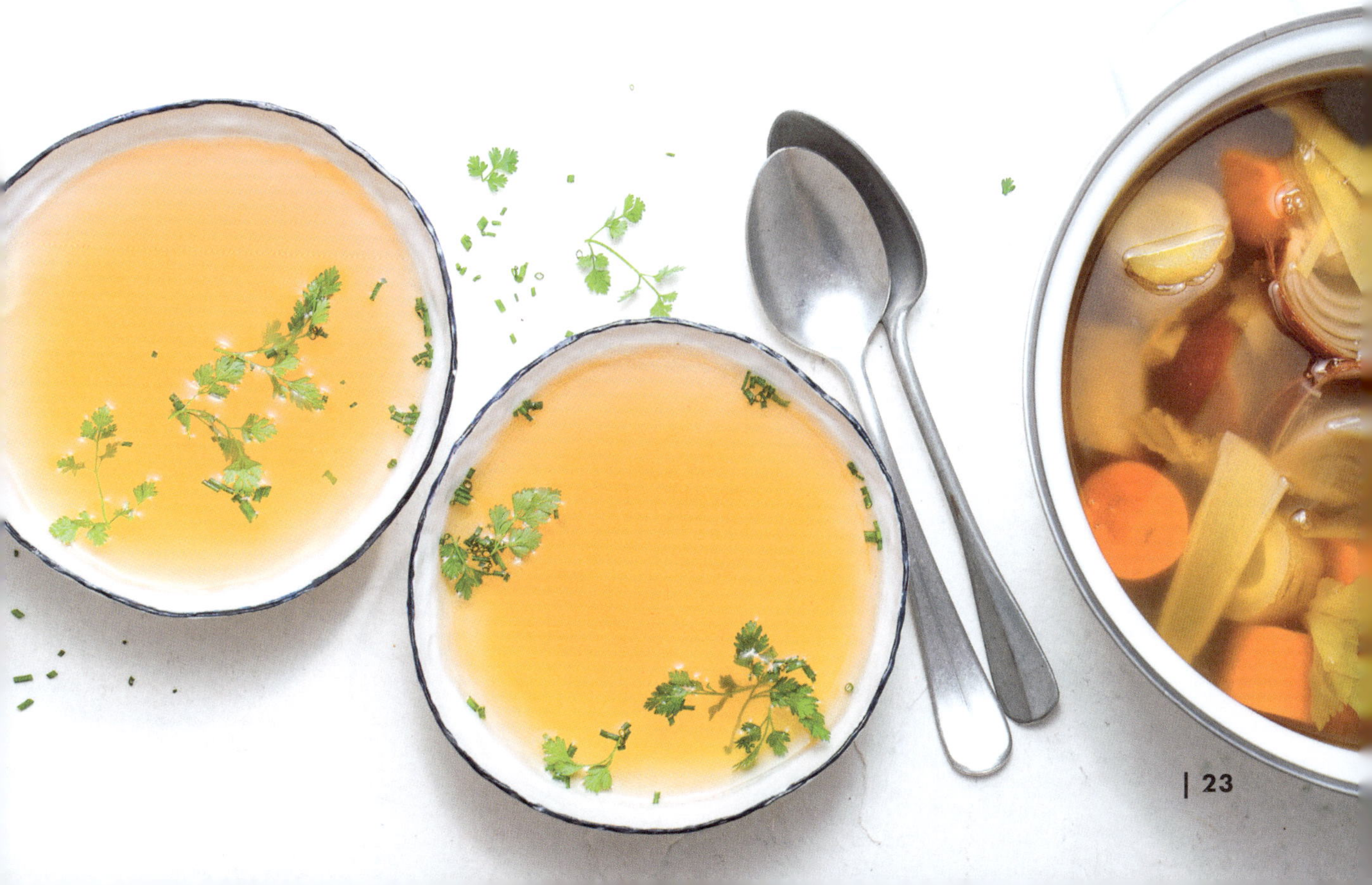

Drinks

As a supplement

Grapefruit, Rosemary and Green Tea Mocktail

MAKES **2 GLASSES**
PREPARATION TIME: **5 MINUTES** • COOKING TIME: **10 MINUTES**
RESTING TIME: **15 MINUTES**

100 ml (3½ fl oz) water
35 g (1½ oz) sugar
3 rosemary sprigs
400ml (14 fl oz) water
1 tablespoon green tea leaves
150 ml (¼ pint) grapefruit juice

1. First, make the syrup. Pour 100 ml (3½ fl oz) water into a saucepan and add the sugar and rosemary sprigs. Bring to the boil and stir until the sugar has dissolved, then turn off the heat and leave to infuse for 15 minutes.
2. Meanwhile, bring 400 ml (14 fl oz) water to the boil. Stir in the green tea and leave to infuse for 5 minutes before straining.
3. Mix the syrup with the grapefruit juice and green tea infusion. Serve chilled over ice, garnished with slices of grapefruit and a fresh rosemary sprigs.

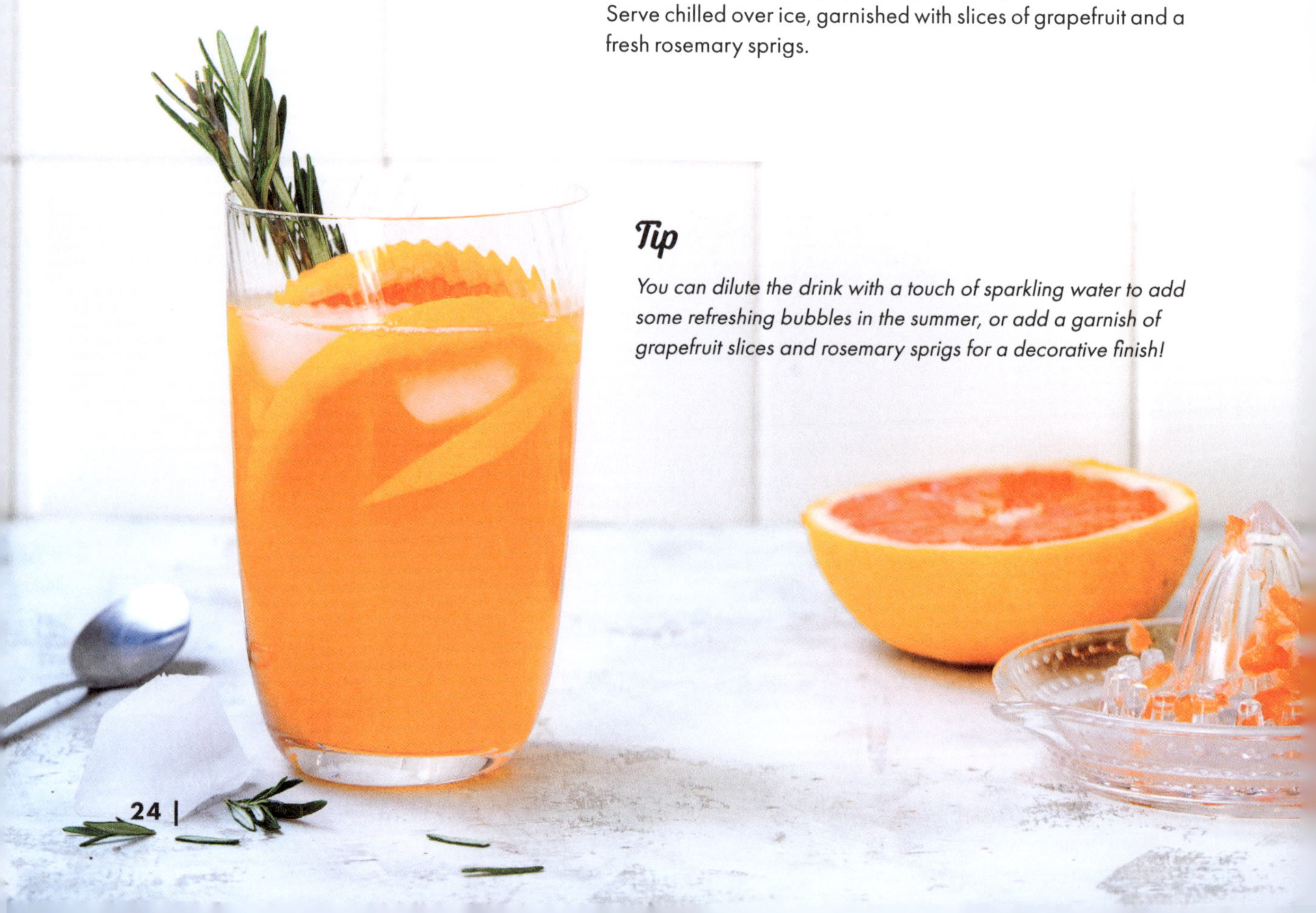

Tip

You can dilute the drink with a touch of sparkling water to add some refreshing bubbles in the summer, or add a garnish of grapefruit slices and rosemary sprigs for a decorative finish!

Drinks

Homemade Kombucha with Red Berries

As a supplement

MAKES **8 GLASSES**
PREPARATION TIME: **10 MINUTES** • COOKING TIME: **5 MINUTES**
RESTING TIME: **3–4 WEEKS**

- 2 litres (3½ pints) water
- 20 g (¾ oz) black or unflavoured green tea leaves
- 180 g (6 oz) sugar
- 1 kombucha mother (scoby)
- 250 g (8 oz) red berries, rinsed and chopped

1. Heat the measured water, add the tea and leave to infuse for about 10 minutes.
2. Add the sugar and stir until completely dissolved, then leave to cool.
3. Once the mixture has reached room temperature, pour into a thoroughly washed jar and add the kombucha mother (scoby), both the solid and liquid parts.
4. Place a cloth over the neck of the jar, secure it with an elastic band and leave to ferment for 2–3 weeks at room temperature (19–32°C/66–90°F) without touching the mixture. After the first 7 days, check that the kombucha mother remains unchanged and shows no signs of mould.
5. At the end of fermentation, remove the kombucha mother using a ladle, then pour the liquid into clean, dry bottles.
6. Divide the berries between the bottles. Close tightly and leave to macerate in the refrigerator for at least 7 days or more.

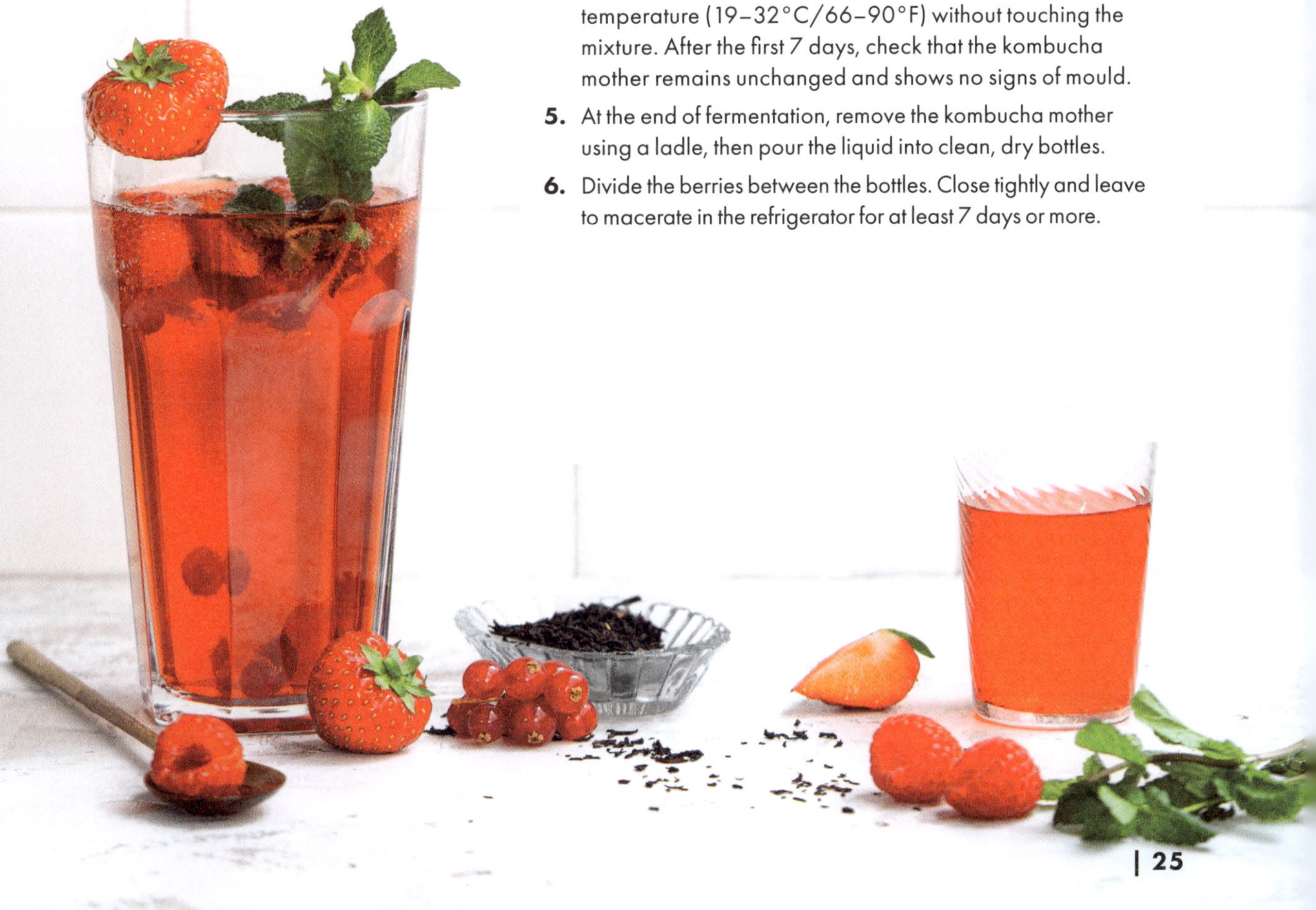

To boost production

Redcurrant, Strawberry and Banana Smoothie

MAKES **4 GLASSES**
PREPARATION TIME: **5 MINUTES**

3 bananas
180 g (6 oz) strawberries
120 g (4 oz) frozen redcurrants, plus extra to garnish
3 tablespoons agave syrup
150 ml (¼ pint) plant-based milk

1. Peel and chop the bananas. Rinse and hull the strawberries.
2. Blitz all the ingredients in a blender until you get a smooth, even texture.
3. Top with extra redcurrants just before serving.

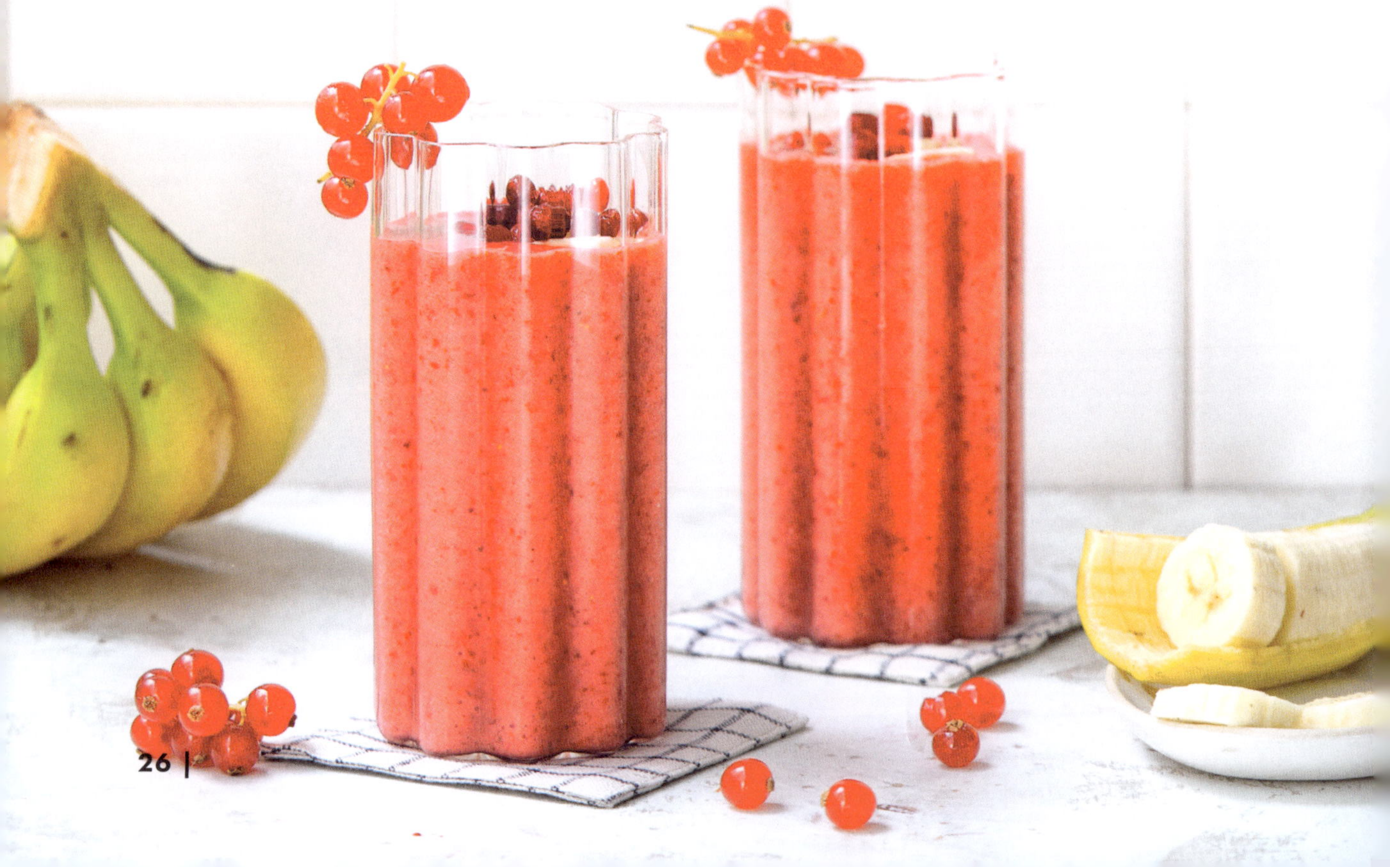

To **boost** production

Pink Beetroot Latte

MAKES **2 GLASSES**
PREPARATION TIME: **10 MINUTES** • COOKING TIME: **10 MINUTES**

½ cooked beetroot
500 ml (17 fl oz) cow's milk or plant-based milk
2 tablespoons honey or agave syrup

FOR TOPPING (OPTIONAL)

150 ml (¼ pint) cow's milk or plant-based milk
½ raw Chioggia beetroot or ½ pink radish, thinly shaved into slices
twist of lemon (optional)

1. Cut the beetroot into chunks and place in a small blender.
2. Heat the milk in a saucepan, then pour it into the blender along with the honey and blitz thoroughly.
3. At the same time, if you like, use a milk frother to froth the milk for topping until it is thick and creamy.
4. Divide the beetroot latte between 2 large glasses and top with the milk froth (if using). Decorate the edge of each glass with a slice of beetroot or radish and top with a twist of lemon, if liked.

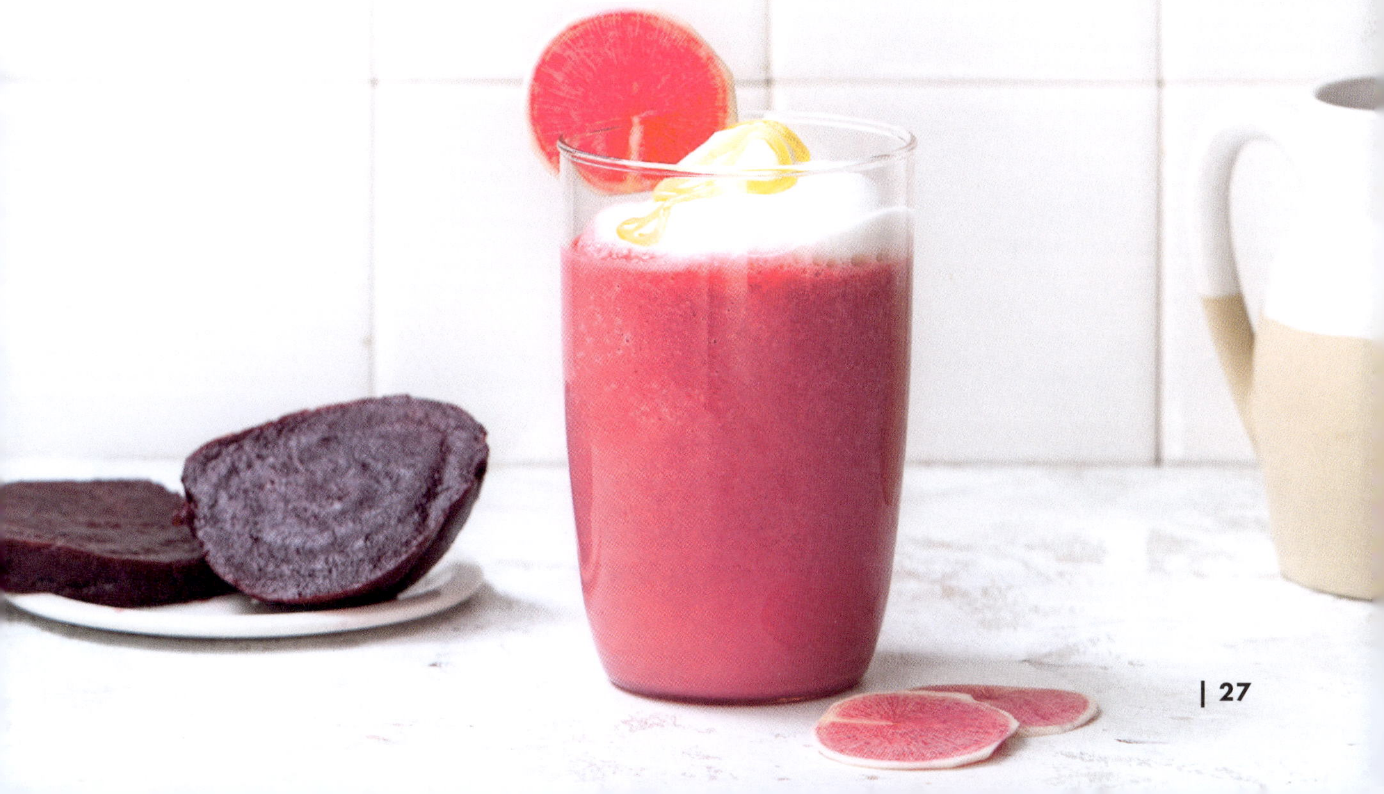

Drinks

Golden Latte

To boost production

MAKES **2 CUPS**
PREPARATION TIME: **10 MINUTES** • COOKING TIME: **5 MINUTES**

½ teaspoon vanilla powder
2 teaspoons ground turmeric
¼ teaspoon ground ginger
½ teaspoon ground cinnamon
500 ml (17fl oz) almond milk
4 tablespoons agave syrup or honey

FOR TOPPING (OPTIONAL)

150 ml (¼ pint) almond milk
150 ml (¼ pint) full-fat milk
½ teaspoon ground turmeric

1. Mix together the vanilla powder, turmeric, ginger and cinnamon.
2. Pour the almond milk into a saucepan and add the agave syrup or honey and the spice mix. Heat gently.
3. For a frothy top, if you like, you can use a milk frother to blend the almond milk and full-fat milk with ground turmeric until creamy in texture.
4. Divide the spiced almond milk between 2 cups and top with the milk froth (if using).

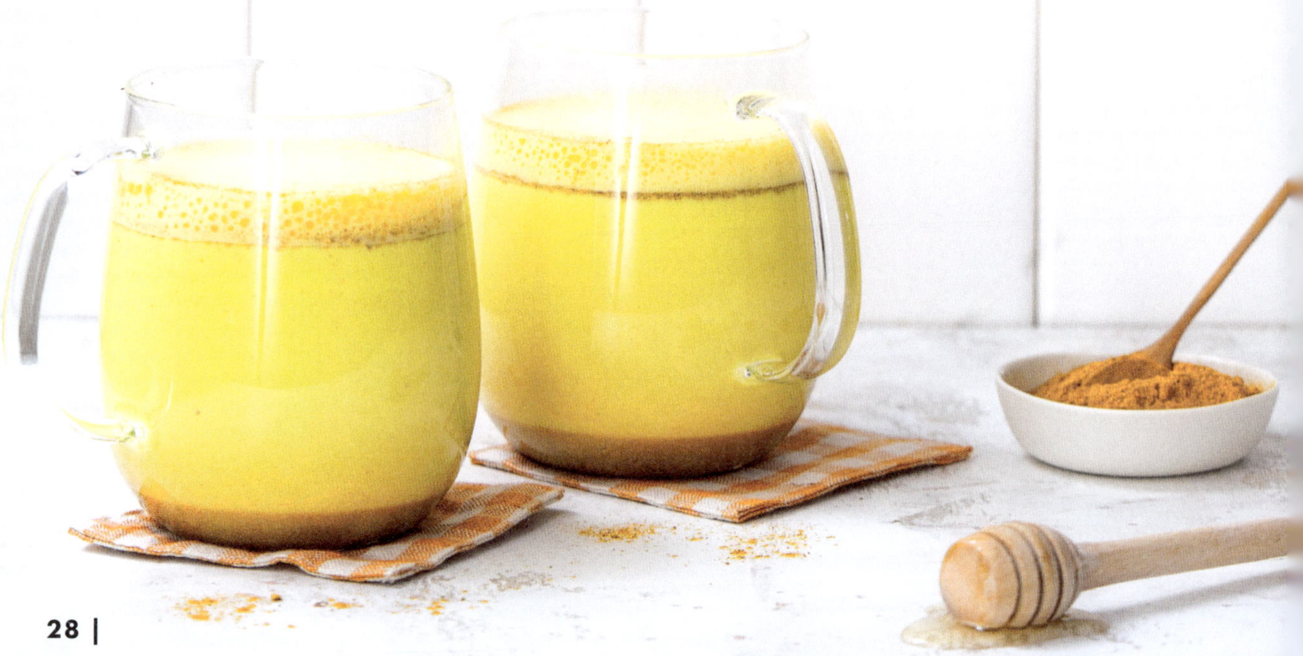

Drinks

Spirulina Latte

To **boost** production

MAKES **2 LARGE CUPS**
PREPARATION TIME: **10 MINUTES**

2 tablespoons honey (optional)
2 tablespoons almond butter
2 tablespoons spirulina powder
500 ml (17 fl oz) milk

FOR TOPPING (OPTIONAL)

150 ml (¼ pint) milk
1 teaspoon spirulina powder, plus extra for sprinkling
8 blueberries

1. Put the honey, almond butter and spirulina powder into a jug.
2. Heat the milk, then pour over the ingredients in the jug. Mix with a whisk.
3. To prepare a topping, if you like, pour the milk and spirulina into a milk frother to make a hot, thick froth.
4. Divide the latte between the 2 cups and top with the milk froth (if using). Sprinkle with the additional spirulina and blueberries.

Tip

You can replace the cow's milk with special 'barista' plant-based milk if you want to achieve a froth that is just as creamy.

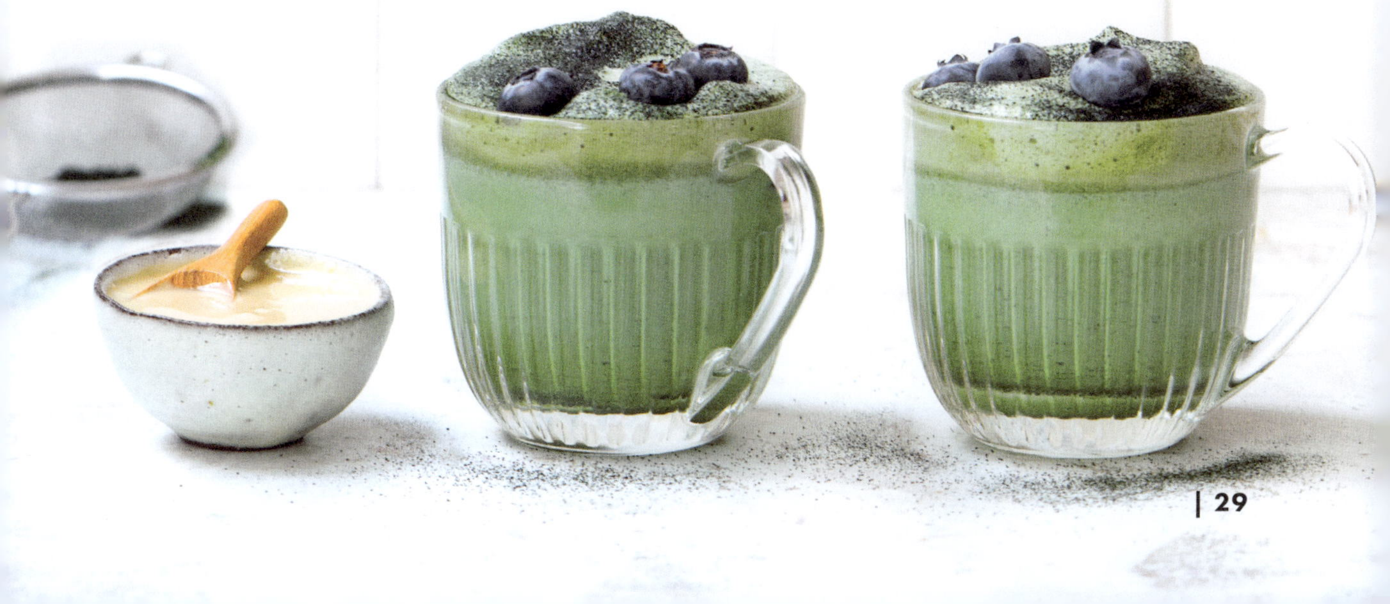

Seasonal Tips

Combine collagen, vitamin C and antioxidants in every meal to enhance the therapeutic effect.

Add turmeric and ginger to your dishes for their anti-inflammatory effects.

Go on a green juice cleanse for a natural boost.

Eat raw, fresh foods, rich in natural enzymes, to maximize collagen assimilation.

Spring Recipes

As a supplement

Light Hibiscus Coconut Jelly

SERVES **6** • PREPARATION TIME: **10 MINUTES** • COOKING TIME: **15 MINUTES**
RESTING TIME: **6 HOURS**

FOR THE HIBISCUS JELLY

6 gelatine leaves
500 ml (17 fl oz) water
2 tablespoons dried hibiscus flowers
80 g (3 oz) caster sugar (optional)

FOR THE COCONUT JELLY

4 gelatine leaves
50 ml (2 fl oz) water
30 g (1 ¼ oz) caster sugar (optional)
200 ml (7 fl oz) coconut milk
pinch of sea salt flakes

1. Start by making the hibiscus jelly: soften the gelatine leaves in a bowl of cold water.
2. Bring the measured water to the boil and add the hibiscus flowers. Turn off the heat, cover the pan and leave to infuse for 10 minutes.
3. Strain and reheat, then add the sugar (if using) and stir until it is dissolved.
4. Remove the pan from the heat, then stir in the softened gelatine until incorporated.
5. Line a high-sided rectangular tray with cling film. Pour in the hibiscus jelly mixture and refrigerate for 4 hours.
6. For the coconut jelly, soften the gelatine leaves as before.
7. Heat the measured water and sugar (if using) in a saucepan until the sugar is fully dissolved. Remove from the heat and add the softened gelatine, coconut milk and salt flakes.
8. Leave to cool before gently pouring the mixture over the chilled hibiscus jelly.
9. Return to the refrigerator for a minimum of 2 hours before cutting into squares.

Tip

If you want to replace the gelatine with a plant-based gelling agent, you can use the following conversion: 4 g (¼ oz) agar agar = about 6 gelatine leaves; 3 (⅙ oz) agar agar = about 4 gelatine leaves.

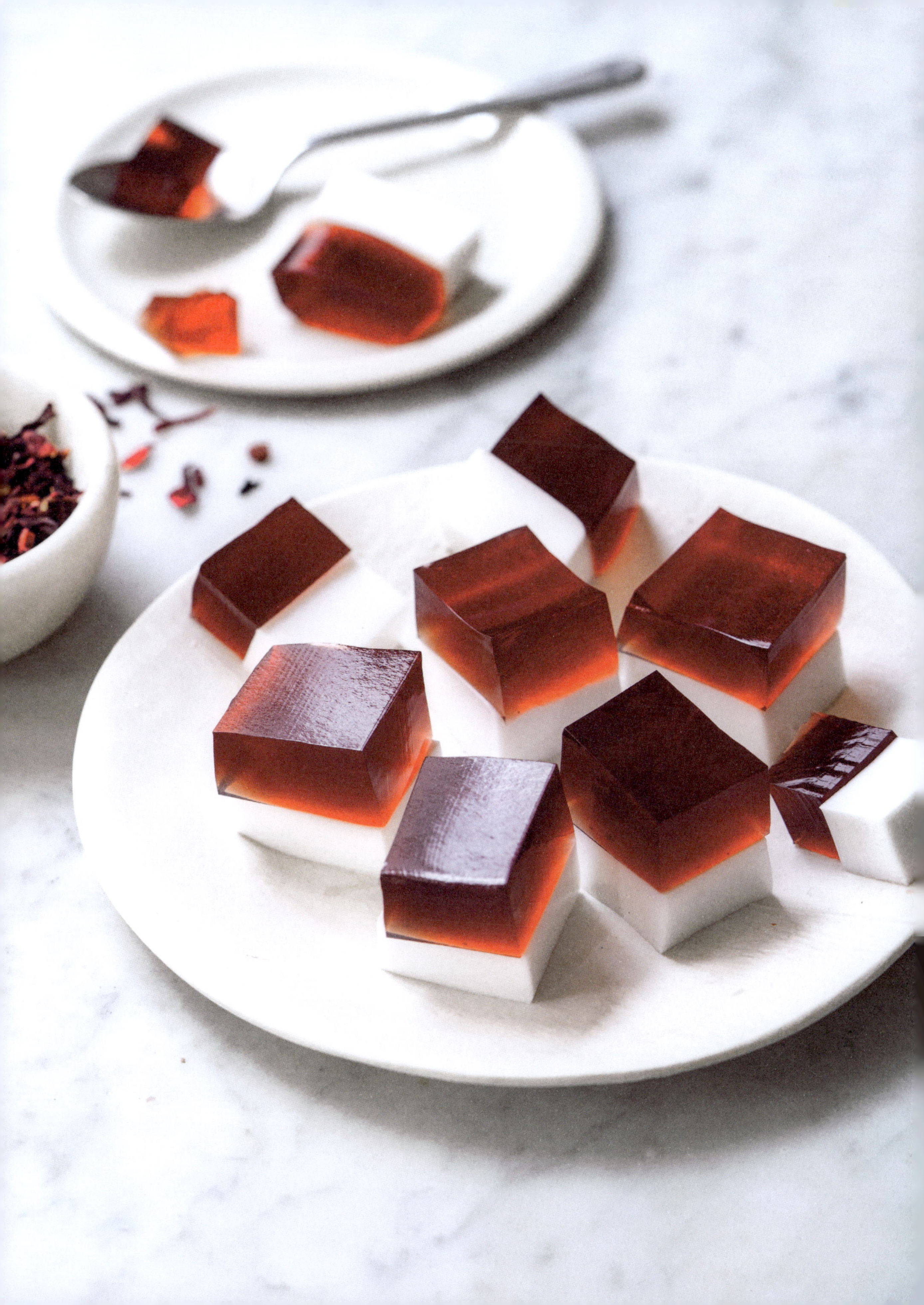

As a supplement

To boost production

7-Hour French-style 'Spoon' Lamb

SERVES **6** • PREPARATION TIME: **15 MINUTES** • COOKING TIME: **6¼–7¼ HOURS**

3 tablespoons olive oil
1 lamb shoulder
4 carrots, peeled and cut into large chunks
3 shallots, peeled and halved lengthways
3 celery sticks, cut into large chunks
1 bulb of garlic, halved widthways
200 ml (7 fl oz) dry white wine
700 ml (24 fl oz) Chicken Stock (see page 16)
1 rosemary sprig
3 thyme sprigs
pinch of coarse sea salt
black pepper, to taste

FOR THE DOUGH SEAL

250 g (8 oz) flour (any kind)
150 ml (¼ pint) water

1. Preheat the oven to 140°C (275°F), Gas Mark 1.
2. Heat the oil in a casserole dish. When hot, brown the meat evenly on all sides, then remove and set aside.
3. Sauté the vegetables in the same oil, including the halved garlic bulb, cut-sides down.
4. Pour in the white wine to deglaze the pan, then return the meat to the pan, taking care to place the vegetables on top of the meat. Pour in the Chicken Stock, then add the herbs and a pinch of coarse salt. Season with black pepper.
5. Mix the flour and water together to make the sealing dough. Seal the lid onto the casserole dish using the dough. Bake in the oven for 6–7 hours.
6. Leave to cool slightly, then break open the dough crust and serve.

Tip

By adding enough liquid (water or stock, depending on what you have to hand) to your casserole dish, you will end up with a good amount of tasty broth. Leftovers can be used in the same way as the other broths and stocks in the plan.

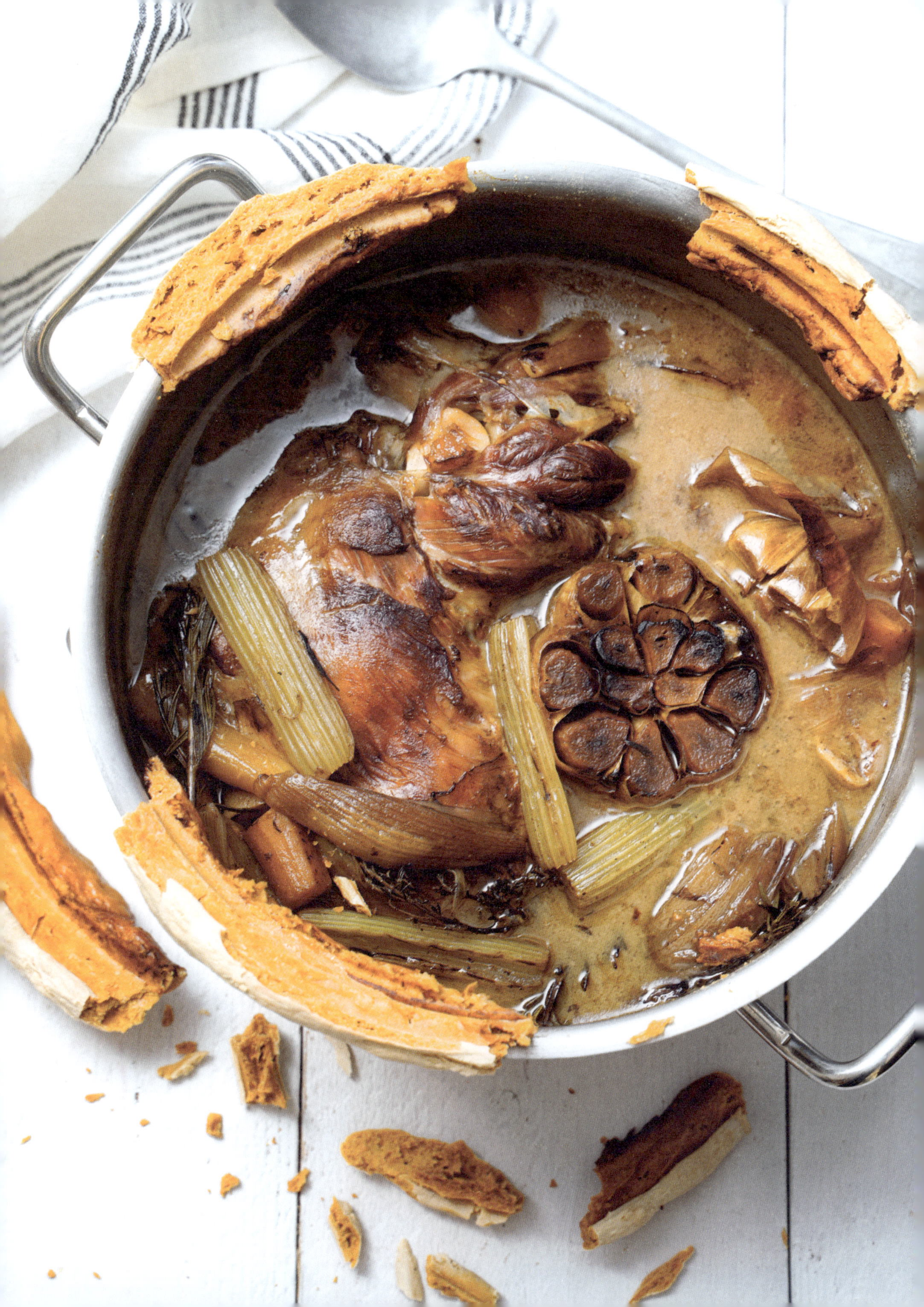

To boost production

Homemade Phô with Meatballs

SERVES **2** • PREPARATION TIME: **15 MINUTES** • COOKING TIME: **10 MINUTES**

Phô Broth (see page 18), hot

FOR THE MEATBALLS

125 g (4 oz) minced beef
3 tablespoons nuoc-mâm (Vietnamese dipping sauce)
½ tablespoon sugar
1 tablespoon cornflour
½ teaspoon baking powder
salt and pepper

TO GARNISH

125 g (4 oz) flat rice noodles
80 g (3 oz) rump steak, very thinly sliced
60 g (2¼ oz) bean sprouts
handful of fresh herbs (mint, Thai basil, coriander etc.)
1 spring onion, finely sliced
1 red chilli, finely sliced (optional)

1. To prepare the meatballs, mix all the ingredients together for 30 seconds. With wet hands, form small meatballs, each about 3 cm (1¼ inches) in diameter.
2. Bring a saucepan of water to the boil and add the meatballs. When they have all risen to the surface, cook them for 7 minutes, then drain.
3. Cook the noodles according to the packet instructions, then drain.
4. Divide the noodles, sliced steak, bean sprouts and meatballs between 2 bowls and pour over the hot broth. Garnish with the herbs, sliced spring onion and chilli (if using).

Tip

You can serve this soup with a wedge of lime to squeeze over the top just before enjoying.

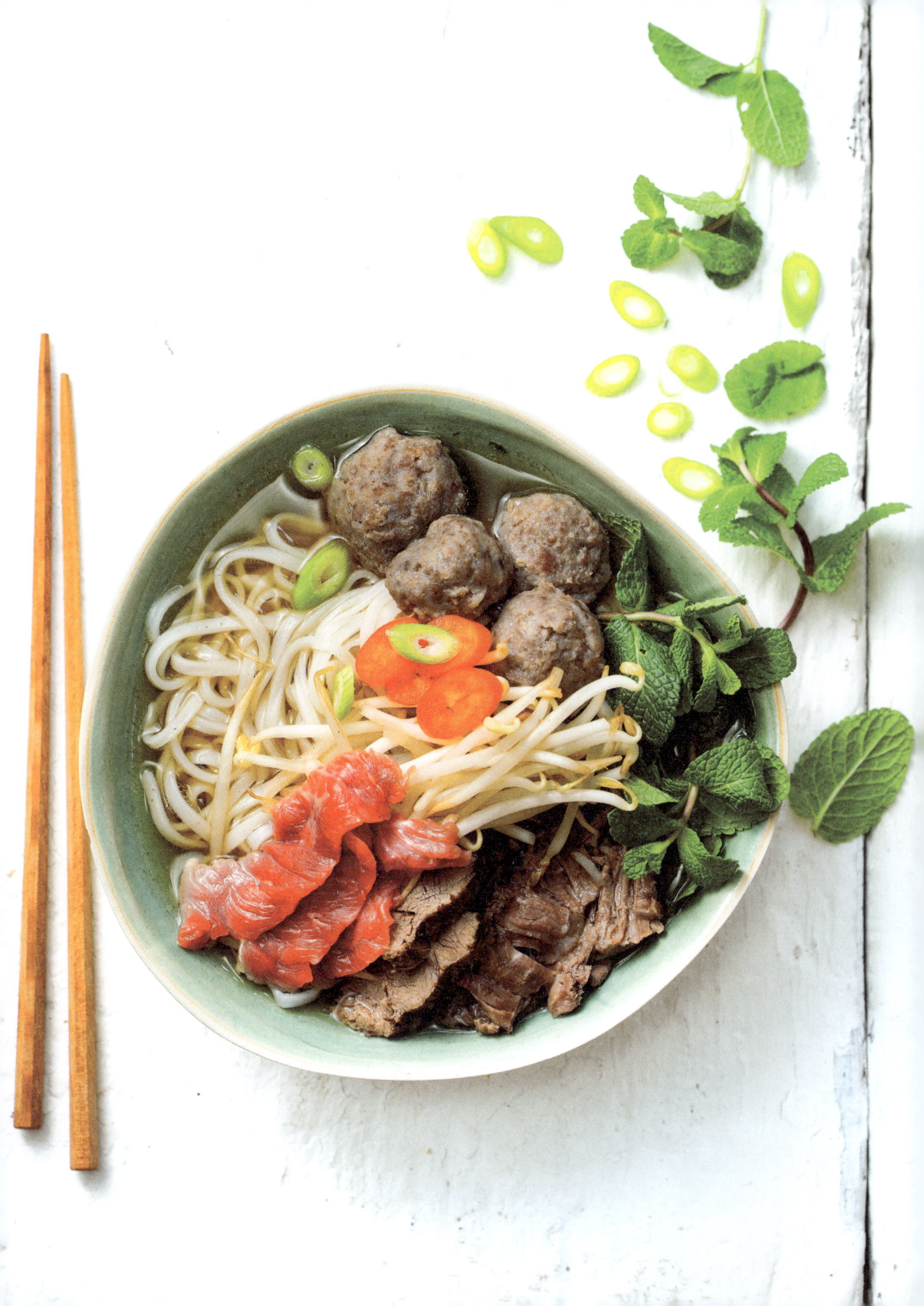

Shredded Chicken Congee

SERVES **2** • PREPARATION TIME: **15 MINUTES** • COOKING TIME: **45 MINUTES**

100 g (3½ oz) rice (ideally jasmine)
1 litre (1¾ pints) Chicken Stock (see page 16)
1 skin-on, bone-in chicken thigh
handful of dried mushrooms
5 g (¼ oz) fresh root ginger, peeled and finely sliced
2 garlic cloves, finely sliced
1 spring onion, finely sliced

TO GARNISH (OPTIONAL)

1 spring onion, finely sliced
chilli oil of choice
2 tablespoons soy sauce
1 teaspoon toasted sesame seeds
aromatic herbs of your choice

1. Wash the rice several times, until the water runs clear, then drain well.
2. Place the rice, Chicken Stock, chicken, dried mushrooms, ginger, garlic and spring onion into a saucepan. Bring to the boil, then cover and cook at a gentle simmer for 45 minutes over a low heat. Stir from time to time.
3. At the end of the cooking time, depending on the desired texture, remove the chicken thigh and break up the grains of rice with a fork to get a creamier porridge-like texture. Shred the chicken meat.
4. Divide the mixture between 2 bowls, adding the shredded meat and garnishes according to taste.

Tip

For a vegetarian version, make the recipe with Vegetable Stock (see page 23) and without the chicken thigh. Add a raw egg yolk to each piping hot bowl just before serving.

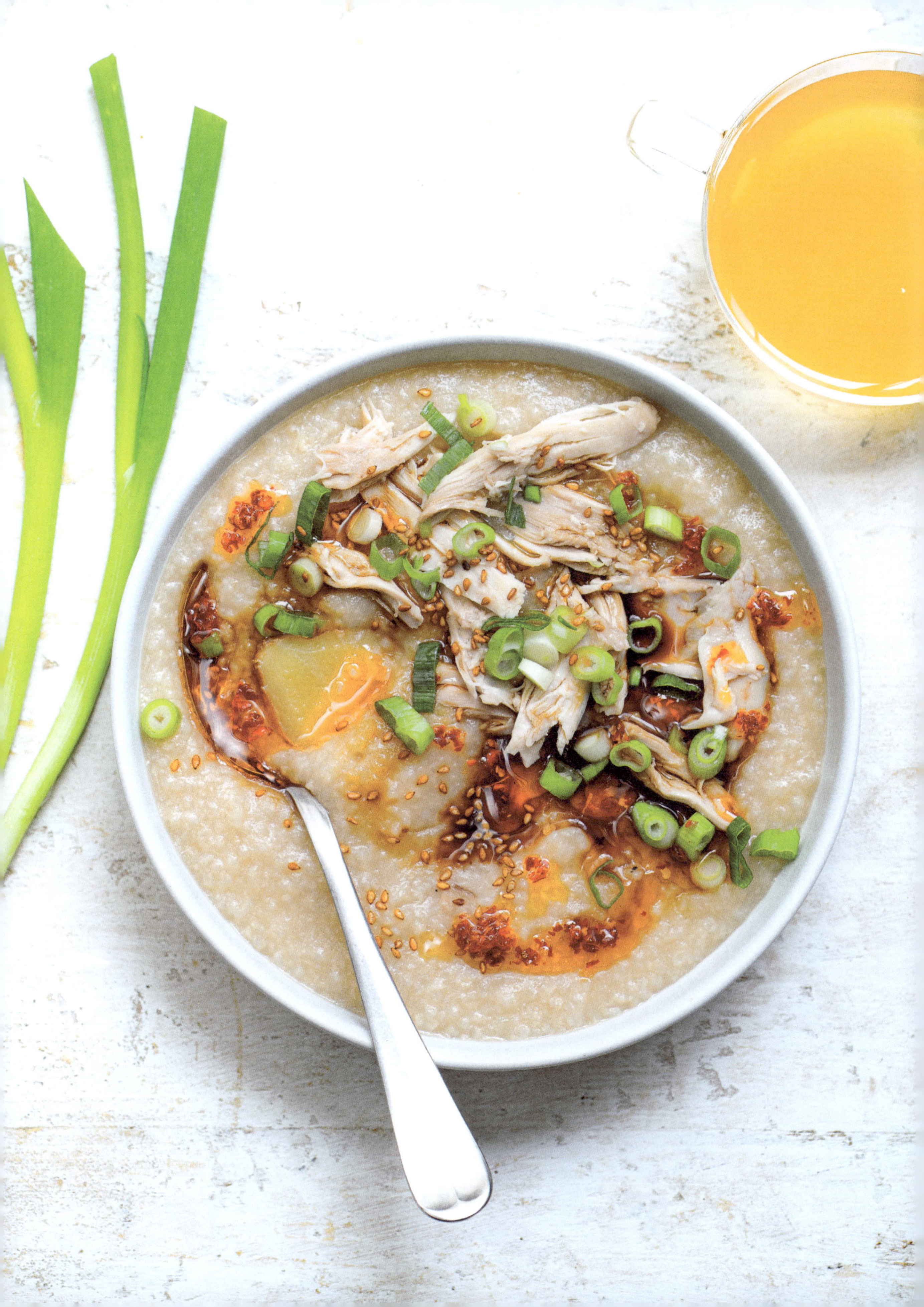

Calves' Liver, Cheesy Asparagus and Mash

To boost production

SERVES **2** • PREPARATION TIME: **10 MINUTES** • COOKING TIME: **45 MINUTES**

500 g (1 lb) firm, waxy potatoes, peeled
50 g (2 oz) butter
handful of chives, chopped
1 bunch of green asparagus
olive oil, for brushing
2 calves' liver slices
4 slices of Tomme de Savoie cheese (about 80 g/3 oz) (alternatively try Reblochon or Comté)
salt and pepper

1. Preheat the grill to hot.
2. Place the potatoes in a saucepan, cover with cold, salted water and bring to the boil. Cook for 20 minutes.
3. Drain the potatoes and mash with a fork, adding 20 g (¾ oz) of the butter and the chives (reserving a little for garnish) until you have a mash. Season with salt and pepper and set aside.
4. Trim the woody ends of the asparagus and place them on a baking sheet. Brush with oil, season with salt and pepper and grill for 10 minutes.
5. Place the slices of cheese on top of the asparagus and grill for a further 5 minutes. Turn off the grill, leaving the cheesy asparagus inside and adding the mashed potato to keep it all warm.
6. Add the remaining butter to a frying pan, then add the calves' liver. Starting from a cold pan, cook over a medium heat for around 7 minutes on each side.
7. Serve the calves' liver with the mashed potato and cheesy baked asparagus, garnished with the reserved chives.

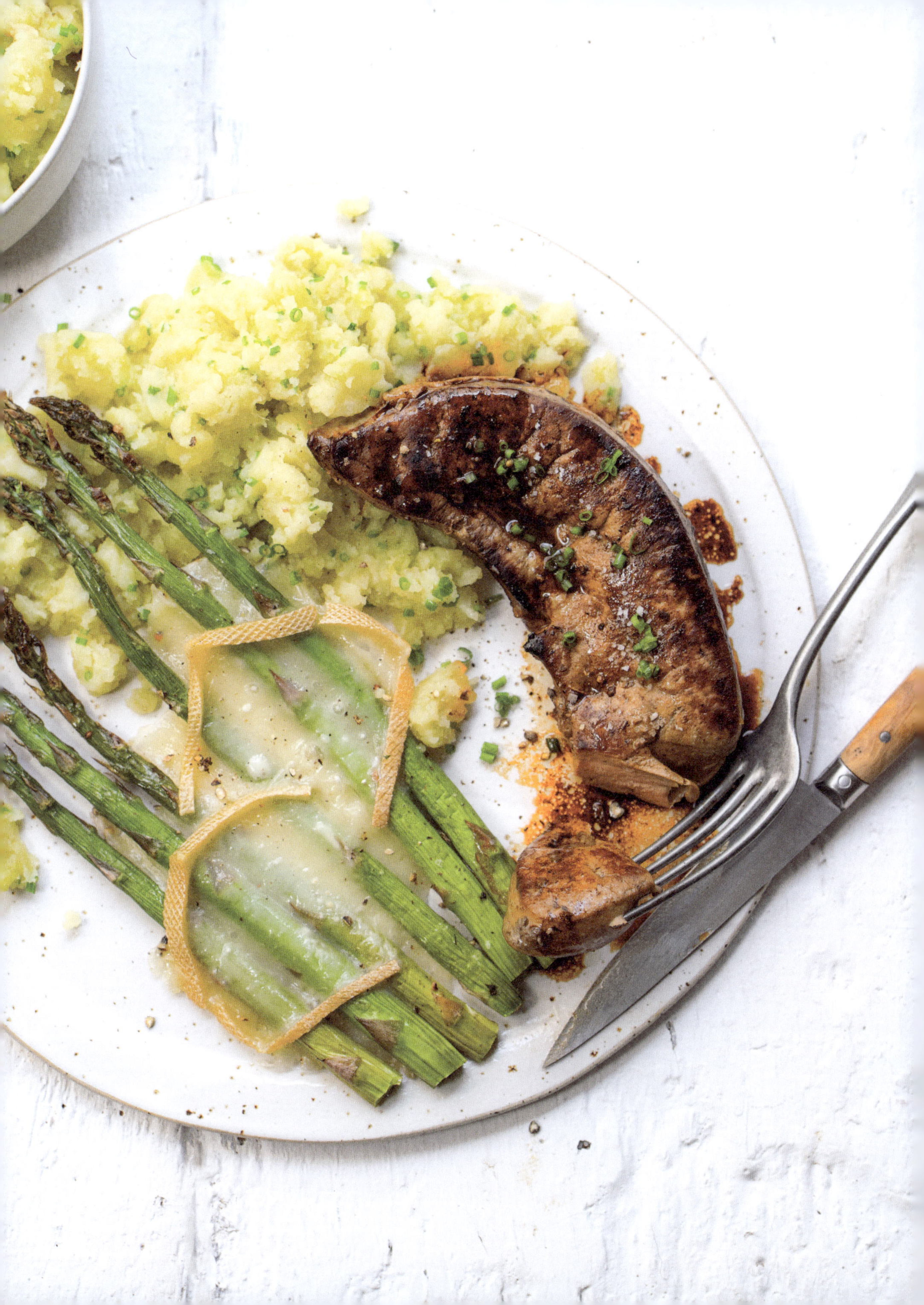

To boost production

Shredded Chicken Noodle Bowl

SERVES **2** • PREPARATION TIME: **20 MINUTES** • COOKING TIME: **30 MINUTES**

500 ml (17 fl oz) Chicken Stock (see page 16)
1 chicken thigh, cooked and shredded
80 g (3 oz) mangetout
1 red pepper, deseeded and diced
125 g (4 oz) wheat noodles
1 small cucumber, thinly sliced
2 small carrots, grated
a few Thai basil leaves
pinch of toasted sesame seeds
1 lime, cut into wedges

FOR THE PEANUT SOY SAUCE

12 g (½ oz) fresh root ginger, peeled and crushed
½ garlic clove, peeled and crushed
120 g (4 oz) unsweetened peanut butter

1. Put the Chicken Stock and shredded chicken into a saucepan and bring to the boil. Cook for 10 minutes to reduce.
2. Meanwhile, cook the mangetout for 5 minutes in a separate pan of boiling water. Refresh in a bowl of cold water. Cut each one diagonally into 2 or 3 pieces. Set aside.
3. Add the diced pepper to the pan of stock and cook for 10 minutes.
4. Add the noodles to the stock pan and cook for 5 minutes (check the cooking time indicated on the packet). Strain the mixture, reserving the stock.
5. Stir all the sauce ingredients together with 150ml (¼ pint) of the reserved Chicken Stock.
6. Mix the noodles with the sauce.
7. Divide the noodles between 2 plates and arrange the shredded chicken meat, pepper and mangetout on the side. Garnish with the cucumber slices, grated carrot, a few Thai basil leaves and a pinch of toasted sesame seeds. Serve with a squeeze of lime.

Tip

For this recipe you can use the leftover chicken from preparing your weekly broth.

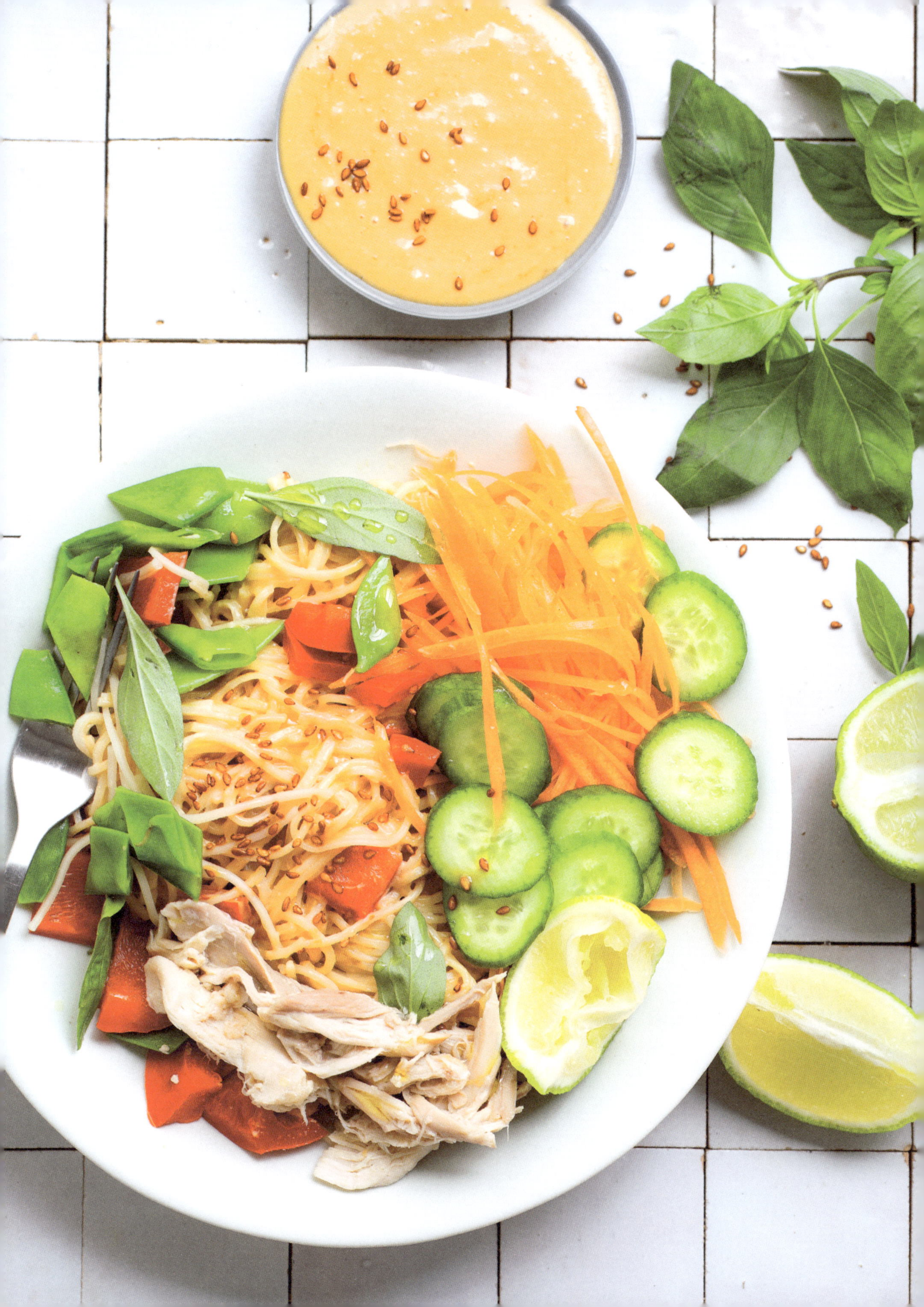

To boost production

Spring Monkfish Stew

SERVES **2** • PREPARATION TIME: **20 MINUTES** • COOKING TIME: **40 MINUTES**

splash of oil
1 spring onion, finely chopped
1 carrot, peeled and cut into thin rounds
150 g (5 oz) button mushrooms (about 3–4 mushrooms), cleaned and quartered
400 ml (14 fl oz) Fish Stock (see page 20)
1 small green courgette, peeled in stripes and cut into thin rounds
1 yellow courgette, peeled in stripes and cut into thin rounds
300 g (10 oz) monkfish fillet, deboned and cut into chunks
100 g (3½ oz) mangetout
30 g (1¼ oz) butter
30 g (1¼ oz) plain flour
100 ml (3½ fl oz) double cream
1 egg yolk
4 chives, finely chopped
juice of ½ lemon
salt and pepper

1. Heat the oil in a casserole dish. When hot, sauté the onion for 2 minutes. Add the carrot and mushrooms and quickly sauté, before pouring in the Fish Stock and adding the courgettes. Cover and simmer for 10 minutes.
2. Add the monkfish and simmer for a further 10 minutes.
3. Meanwhile, cook the mangetout in salted boiling water for 5 minutes. Drain and refresh in cold water to stop the cooking process.
4. Using a slotted spoon, carefully transfer the cooked vegetables and fish to a serving dish, along with the mangetout, and keep warm. Reserve the stock.
5. In a small saucepan, melt the butter, then add the flour and stir to form a roux. Whisking all the time over a medium heat, gradually add the Fish Stock and cream until everything is well combined.
6. Remove the sauce from the heat and stir in the egg yolk, chives and lemon juice.
7. Pour the creamy sauce over the vegetables and fish, season with salt and pepper, then serve.

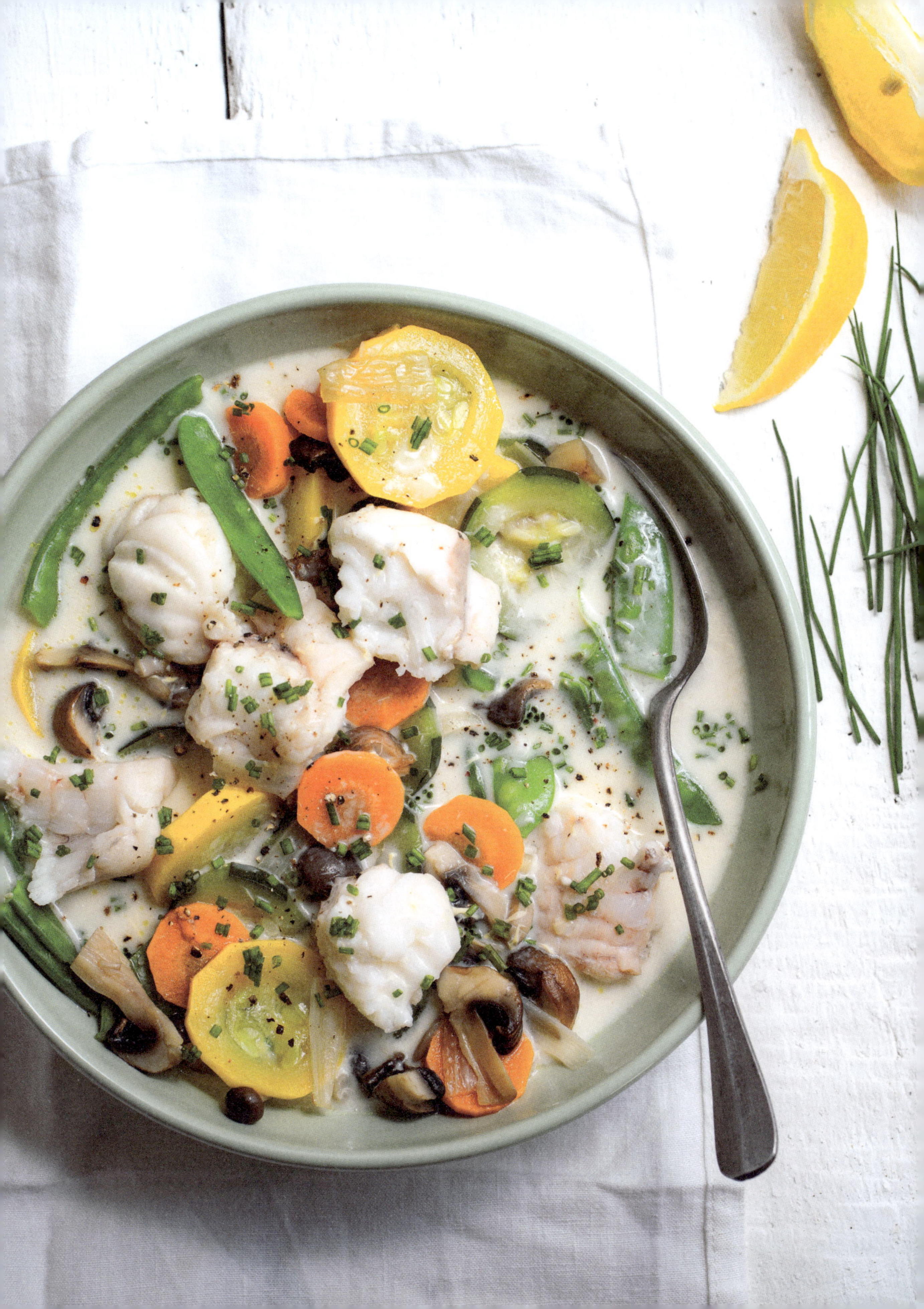

COLLAGEN THERAPY • SPRING

For radiant skin and a burst of energy

Here we are going to prioritize the sources of Type I collagen, specifically targeting skin, tendons and bone. Spring is the ideal season to revitalize the skin and stimulate energy after winter. The emphasis is on elimination of toxins, with antioxidants and vitamin C to strengthen collagen and support cellular regeneration.

AIM

To stimulate collagen production for radiant skin and new-found vitality.

To boost production

KEY NUTRIENTS

To stimulate collagen production naturally, some essential cofactors are required.

- **Vitamin C** (citrus fruit, red berries, peppers, parsley and broccoli)
- **Zinc and copper** (oysters, seeds, dark chocolate, cashew nuts, sunflower seeds, lean red meat)
- **Omega-3 fatty acids** (oily fish, avocado, flaxseed)
- **Antioxidants** (green tea, berries, raw cacao, carrots, turmeric)

As a supplement

KEY FOODS

The following foods contain bioavailable collagen for the skin, hair and nails.

Fish, including the skin and bones (salmon, sardines, mackerel)

Chicken (skin and cartilage)

Bone broth (beef, chicken, fish)

Egg white (rich in proline, a precursor to collagen)

Pork rind (baked, jellied, in homemade pâté)

Natural gelatine and collagen powder

	DAY 1	DAY 2
BREAKFAST	Nut, Seed and Goji Berry Cereal Bar • see page 60 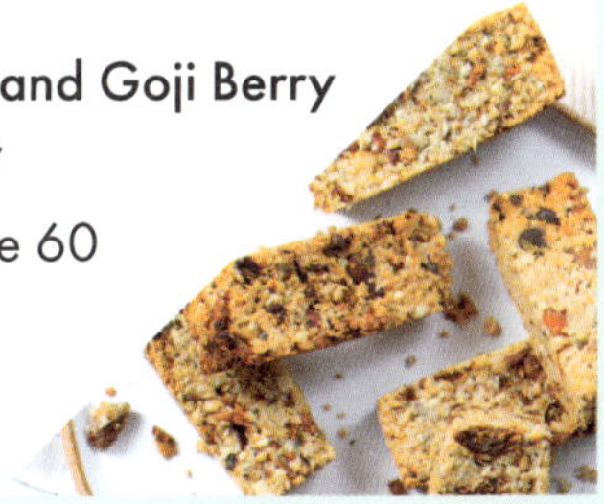	Banana Pancakes • see page 92 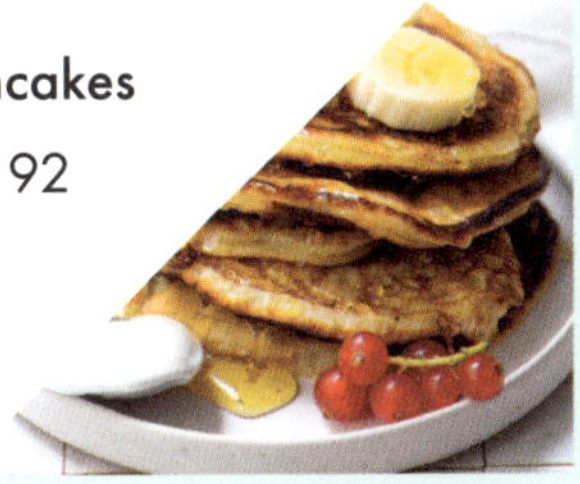
LUNCH	Shredded Chicken Noodle Bowl • see page 42 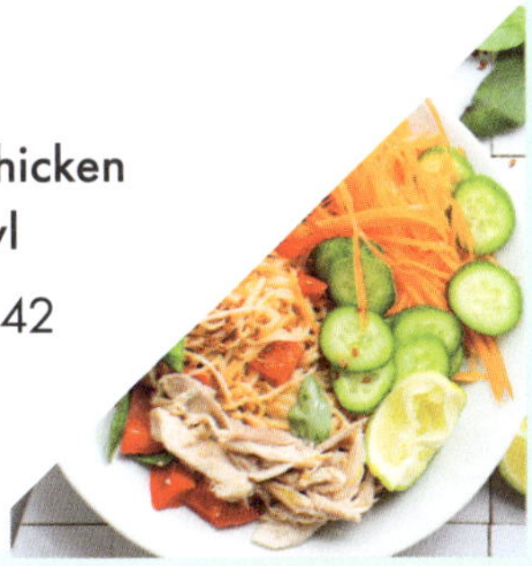	**Grilled salmon salad:** mix some salmon (skin included) with avocado, citrus fruit and a vinaigrette of your choice, for a good dose of vitamin C and Omega-3 fatty acids
SNACK	Light Hibiscus Coconut Jelly • see page 32 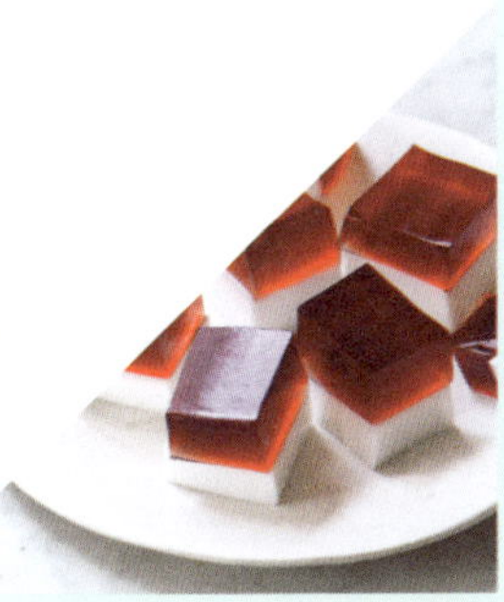	**Collagen smoothie:** blend 1 pot of natural yogurt (calcium, probiotics), ½ banana, a handful of red berries and 1 tablespoon chia seeds
DINNER	**Chicken Stock** with added seeds and small pasta shapes • see page 16 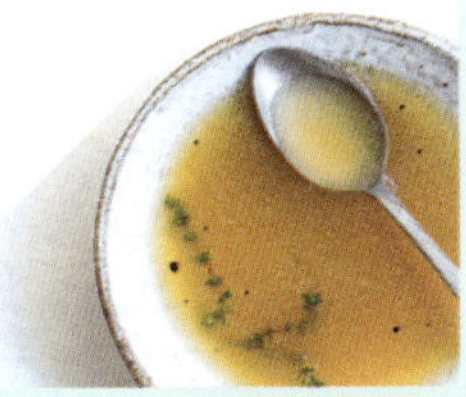	Super-Green Soup • see page 52 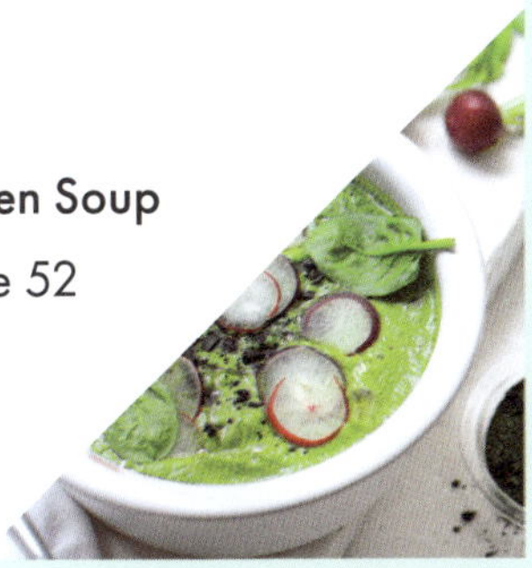

Prawn Tom Kha Soup

As a supplement

To boost production

SERVES **2** • PREPARATION TIME: **10 MINUTES** • COOKING TIME: **35 MINUTES**

1 tablespoon oil
300 g (10 oz) frozen, raw, shelled prawns
1 onion, finely chopped
1 lemongrass stalk, lightly crushed
1 tablespoon red curry paste
1.5 litres (2½ pints) Thai-style Prawn Broth (see page 21)
200 g (7 oz) mushrooms, cleaned and sliced (depending on size and type)
250 ml (8 fl oz) coconut cream
1 green tomato, sliced
1 tablespoon brown sugar
1 spring onion, finely chopped

1. Heat the oil in a saucepan. When hot, sauté the prawns and the onion for 2 minutes.
2. Tie the lemongrass stalk in a knot and add to the pan along with the curry paste and the broth. Cook for 5 minutes, then remove the prawns with a slotted spoon and set aside.
3. Add the mushrooms to the pan and cook for a further 20 minutes.
4. Pour in the coconut cream, return the prawns to the pan, add the tomato and brown sugar and cook for 5 minutes.
5. Serve garnished with the chopped spring onion.

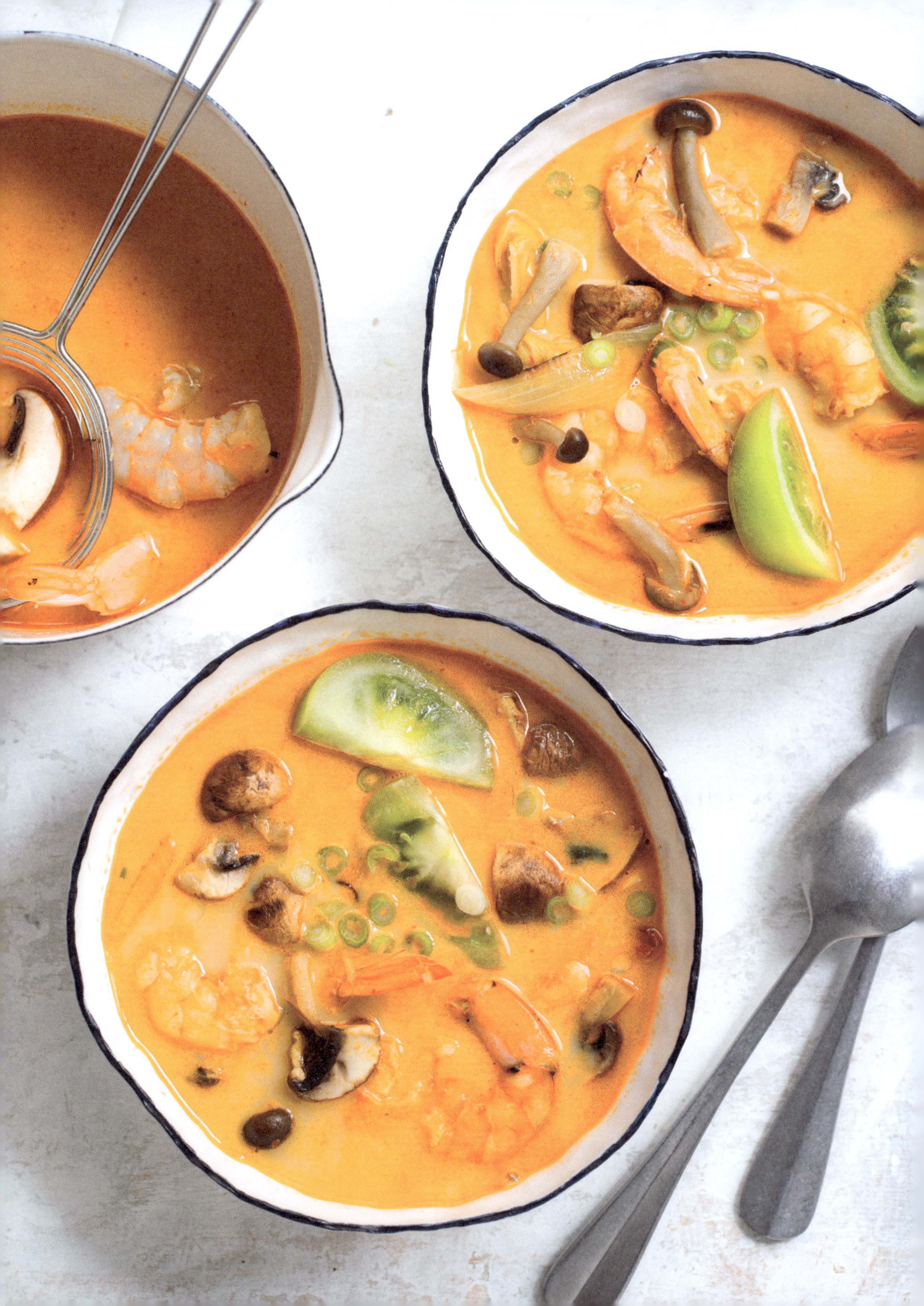

As a supplement

To boost production

Salmon and Rice Salad with Green Vegetables

SERVES **2** • PREPARATION TIME: **10 MINUTES** • COOKING TIME: **40 MINUTES**

2 boneless, skinless salmon steaks
¼ bunch of dill, finely chopped
1 teaspoon fennel seeds, crushed
1 teaspoon pink peppercorns, crushed
2 tablespoons olive oil
6 asparagus spears
3 kale leaves, stalks removed
80 g (3 oz) brown rice
½ cucumber (or 1 small Lebanese cucumber), thinly sliced
1 teaspoon nutritional yeast
½ lemon, cut into wedges
salt and pepper

FOR THE CAESAR-STYLE SAUCE

30 g (1¼ oz) mayonnaise
70 g (2¾ oz) Skyr or Greek-style yogurt
juice of ½ lemon
60 g (2¼ oz) Parmesan cheese, grated
1 garlic clove, crushed
2 anchovies, finely chopped
4 tarragon sprigs (or chives), finely chopped

1. Cut the salmon into cubes and mix it with the dill, fennel seeds, pink peppercorns and olive oil.
2. Trim the woody ends of the asparagus, then cook for 6 minutes in a steamer.
3. Add the kale leaves to the steamer and cook for a further 5 minutes.
4. Heat a grill pan until hot, then grill the salmon pieces for 5 minutes, turning as needed.
5. Cook the brown rice according to the packet instructions.
6. To make the sauce, combine all the ingredients in a small bowl.
7. Mix the cooked rice with the kale and divide between 2 bowls. Top with the pieces of grilled salmon, asparagus and sliced cucumber. Season with salt and pepper and sprinkle some nutritional yeast over the top. Serve with the sauce and lemon wedges on the side.

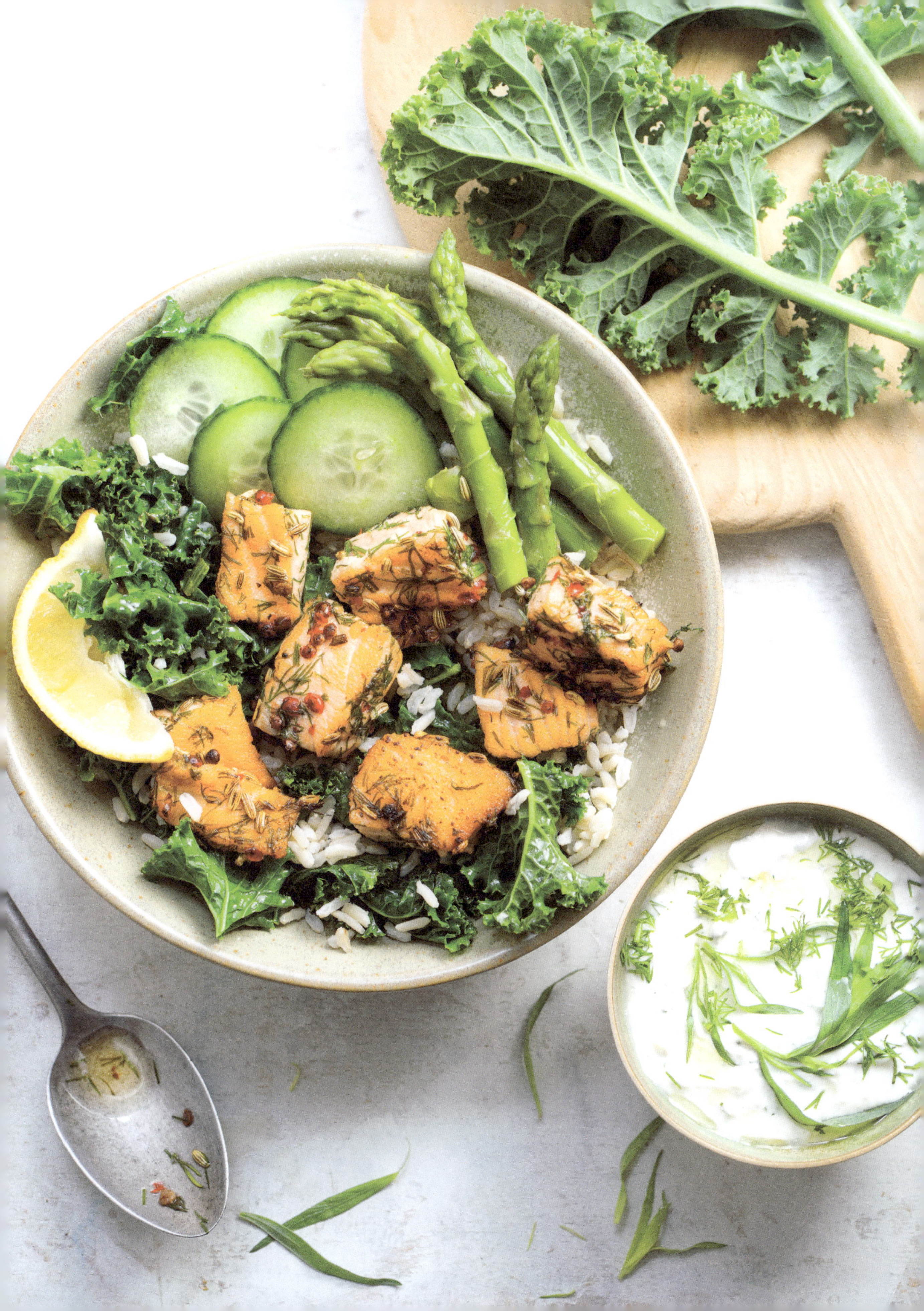

To boost production

Super-Green Soup

SERVES **2** • PREPARATION TIME: **25 MINUTES** • COOKING TIME: **25 MINUTES**

splash of oil
1 onion, roughly chopped
1 garlic clove, roughly chopped
1 green courgette, diced
½ head of broccoli, cut into florets
1 leek top (green part), roughly chopped
200 g (7 oz) green beans
1 bundle of green asparagus (optional), woody ends trimmed, then cut into short lengths
750 ml (1 ¼ pints) Vegetable Stock (see page 23)
pinch of coarse salt
60 g baby spinach (or kale)
½ avocado
pinch of green spirulina powder
pinch of ground black pepper

FOR THE TOPPINGS

4 radishes, thinly sliced
pinch of green spirulina powder
extra baby spinach leaves

1. Preheat the oven to 180°C (350°F), Gas Mark 4.
2. Heat the oil in a large saucepan over a medium heat. When hot, sauté the onion and garlic for 2–3 minutes, then add the courgette, broccoli florets, leek, green beans and asparagus (if using). Cover with stock and add a pinch of coarse salt. Cook at a simmer for 10 minutes.
3. Add the baby spinach to the pan and cook for a further 5 minutes. Pierce the vegetables with a knife to check whether they are cooked.
4. When ready, transfer everything to a blender along with the avocado flesh, spirulina and a pinch of ground pepper. Blend until smooth.
5. Serve in bowls, sprinkled with the toppings.

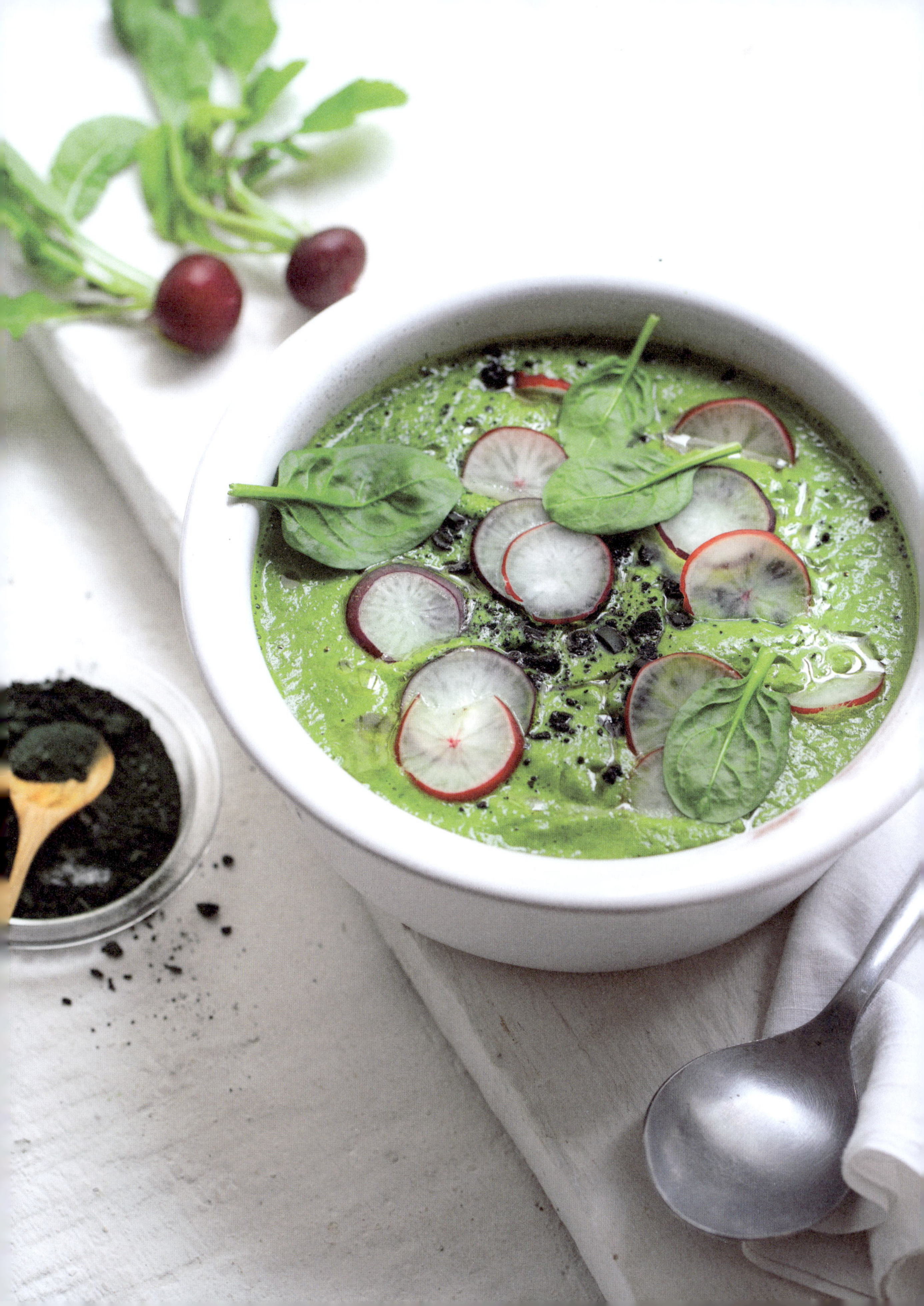

To **boost** production

Green Bean, Hazelnut and Strawberry Salad

SERVES **2** • PREPARATION TIME: **15 MINUTES** • COOKING TIME: **15 MINUTES**

220 g (7½ oz) green beans, trimmed
30 g (1¼ oz) hazelnuts
250 g (8 oz) strawberries
70 g (2¾ oz) feta cheese, crumbled
2 tarragon sprigs, finely chopped
6 chives, finely chopped
1 spring onion, finely sliced
salt and pepper

FOR THE VINAIGRETTE

2 tablespoons cider vinegar (or lemon juice)
2 tablespoons hazelnut oil

1. Preheat the oven to 150°C (300°F), Gas Mark 2.
2. Place the green beans in a large saucepan of salted boiling water and cook for 10–12 minutes, then drain and drop into a large bowl of cold water to stop the cooking process.
3. Meanwhile, spread the hazelnuts over a baking sheet and roast in the oven for 15 minutes. Rub the hazelnuts while still hot in a tea towel to remove as much skin as possible, then roughly chop them.
4. Mash half of the strawberries with a fork, then strain so you are left with just the juice. Combine the juice with the vinegar (or lemon juice) and hazelnut oil to make the vinaigrette.
5. Chop the remaining strawberries.
6. In a large bowl, combine the beans, chopped strawberries, crumbled feta, hazelnuts, tarragon, chives and spring onion. Dress with the vinaigrette, season with salt and pepper and serve immediately.

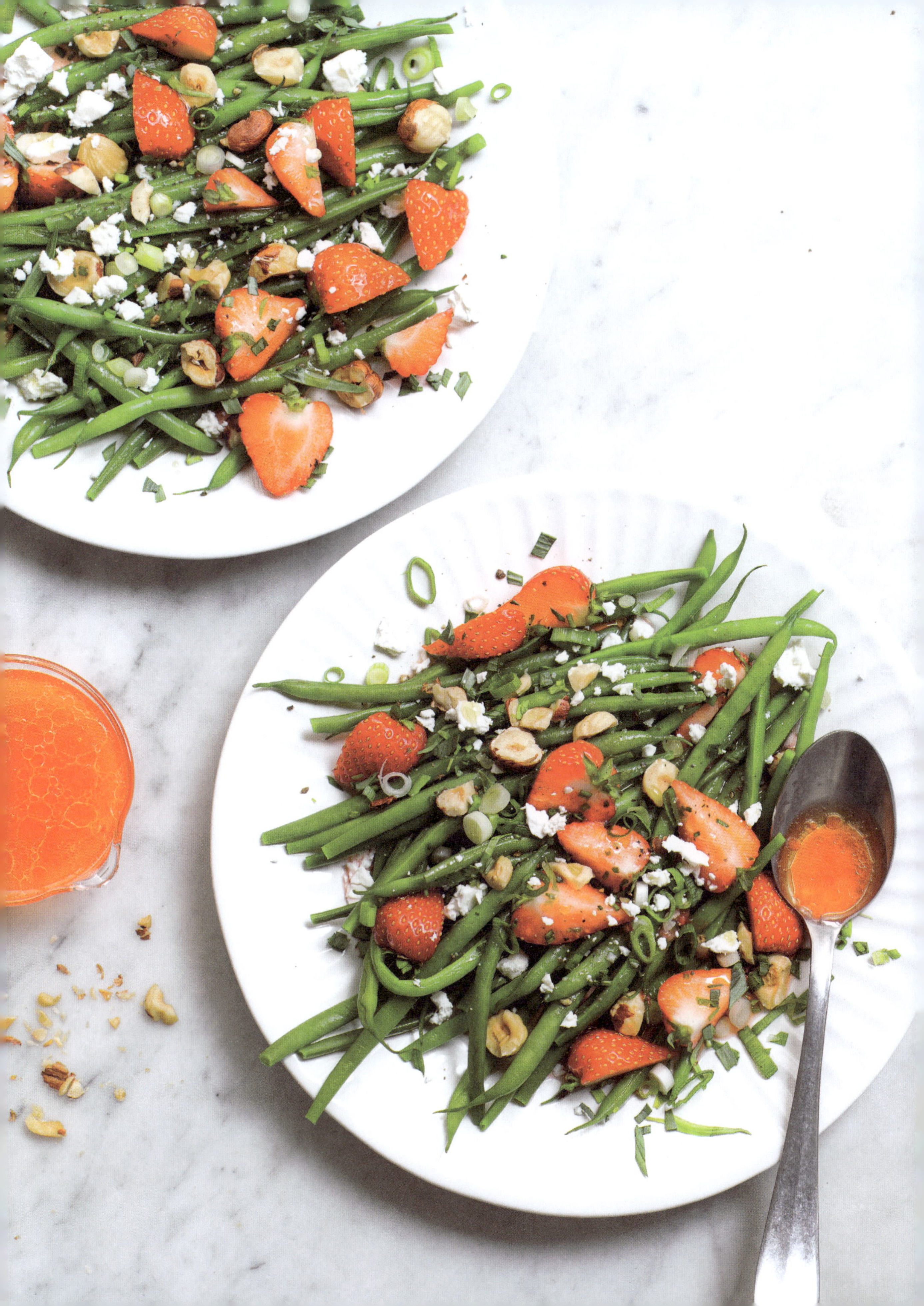

To boost production

Vegetarian Burger

SERVES **2** • PREPARATION TIME: **20 MINUTES** • COOKING TIME: **15 MINUTES**

FOR THE BURGER PATTIES

100 g (3½ oz) button mushrooms, roughly chopped

35 g (1½ oz) bread, diced

50 g (2 oz) canned kidney beans (drained)

½ teaspoon ground cumin

4 parsley sprigs, finely chopped

40 g (1¾ oz) canned sweetcorn (drained)

salt and pepper

1 tablespoon sunflower oil, for cooking

FOR THE SAUCE

¼ onion, finely chopped

50 g (2 oz) mayonnaise

1 teaspoon yellow mustard

2 teaspoons tomato ketchup

pinch of smoked paprika

TO SERVE

2 burger buns, halved

20 g (¾ oz) softened butter

4 burger cheese slices

handful of rocket leaves

1 tomato, thinly sliced

½ avocado, thinly sliced

sprinkle of red onion, finely chopped

1. To make the burgers, blitz the mushrooms, bread, kidney beans, cumin and some salt and pepper in a food processor until smooth. Add the parsley and sweetcorn and mix well. Shape the mixture into 2 patties.
2. To make the sauce, combine all the ingredients in a bowl.
3. Spread the inside of the burger buns with the soft butter and toast them in a hot pan for 3 minutes. Set aside.
4. Heat the sunflower oil in a frying pan. When hot, add the patties and fry for 3 minutes on each side. Place a slice of burger cheese on top of each patty, then turn down the heat and cover. Cook for a further 5 minutes until the cheese has melted.
5. Spread the sauce on the buns and fill with the rocket, tomato and burger patties. Top with the avocado slices and the other half of the bun.

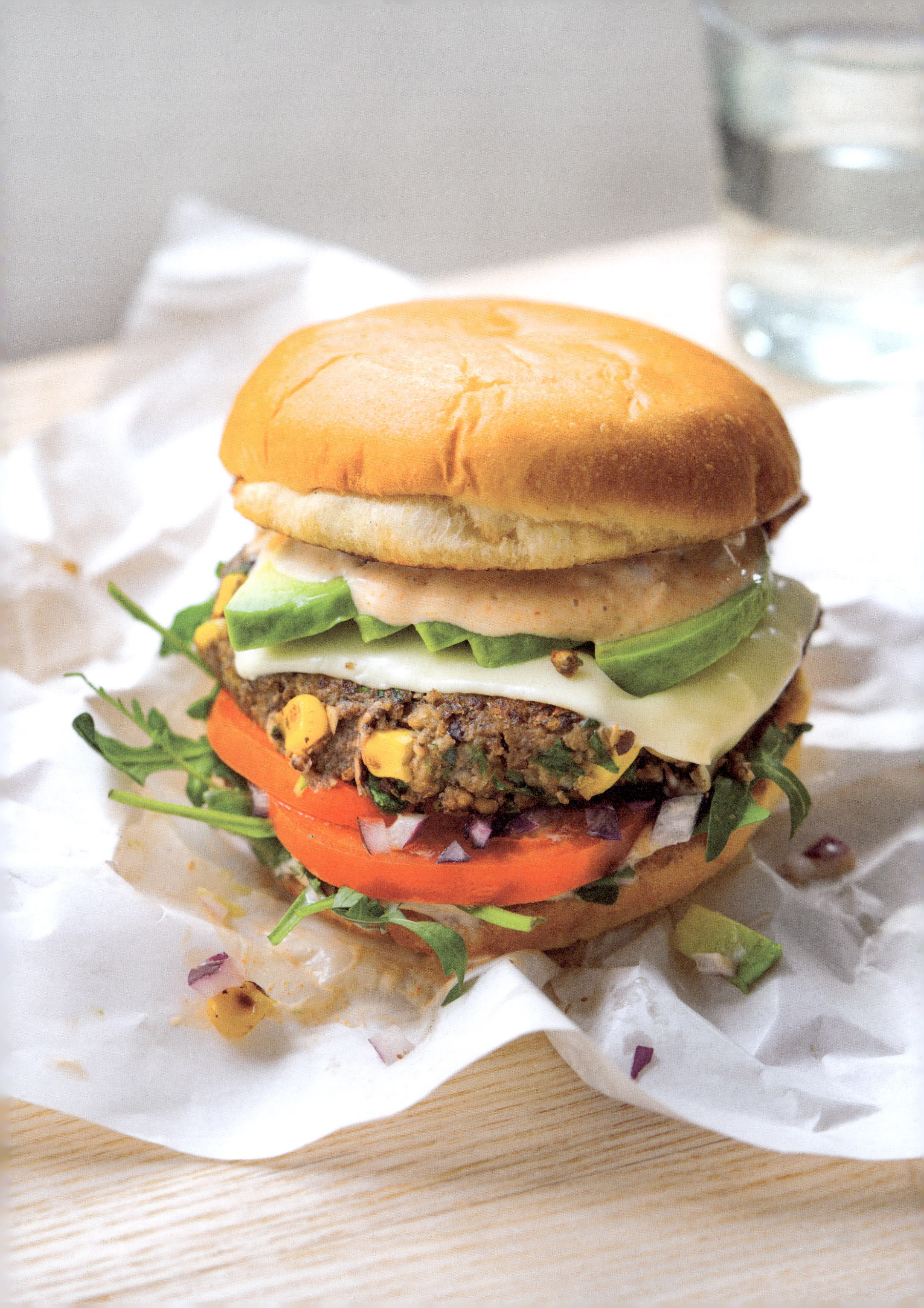

To boost production

Savoury Steamed Egg Flan

SERVES **2** • PREPARATION TIME: **10 MINUTES** • COOKING TIME: **25 MINUTES**

4 fresh shiitake mushrooms (or button mushrooms, porcini etc.), thinly sliced
60 g (2¼ oz) frozen broad beans (or edamame)
2 tablespoons water
4 eggs
pinch of fine salt
Dashi (see page 22) or stock of choice, at room temperature – you will need 1½ times the volume of stock to the volume of eggs

TO SERVE

1 teaspoon sesame oil
3 tablespoons soy sauce
4 coriander sprigs, finely chopped
1 spring onion, finely sliced

1. Place the sliced mushrooms in a frying pan with the broad beans and measured water. Cover and steam over a low heat for 10 minutes.
2. Meanwhile, beat the eggs with the salt and check their volume. Add the required amount of dashi or stock and mix well.
3. Divide the steamed vegetables between 2 ramekins or heatproof bowls. Using a sieve to remove any lumps, pour the egg mixture over the top.
4. Fill a saucepan with boiling water and place a steamer basket over the top. Place the ramekins or bowls in the basket, cover and steam for 15 minutes, checking all the time that the heat is not too high.
5. Carefully remove from the steamer and cut the flans in a grid pattern. Pour over the sesame oil and soy sauce, then top with coriander and spring onion.

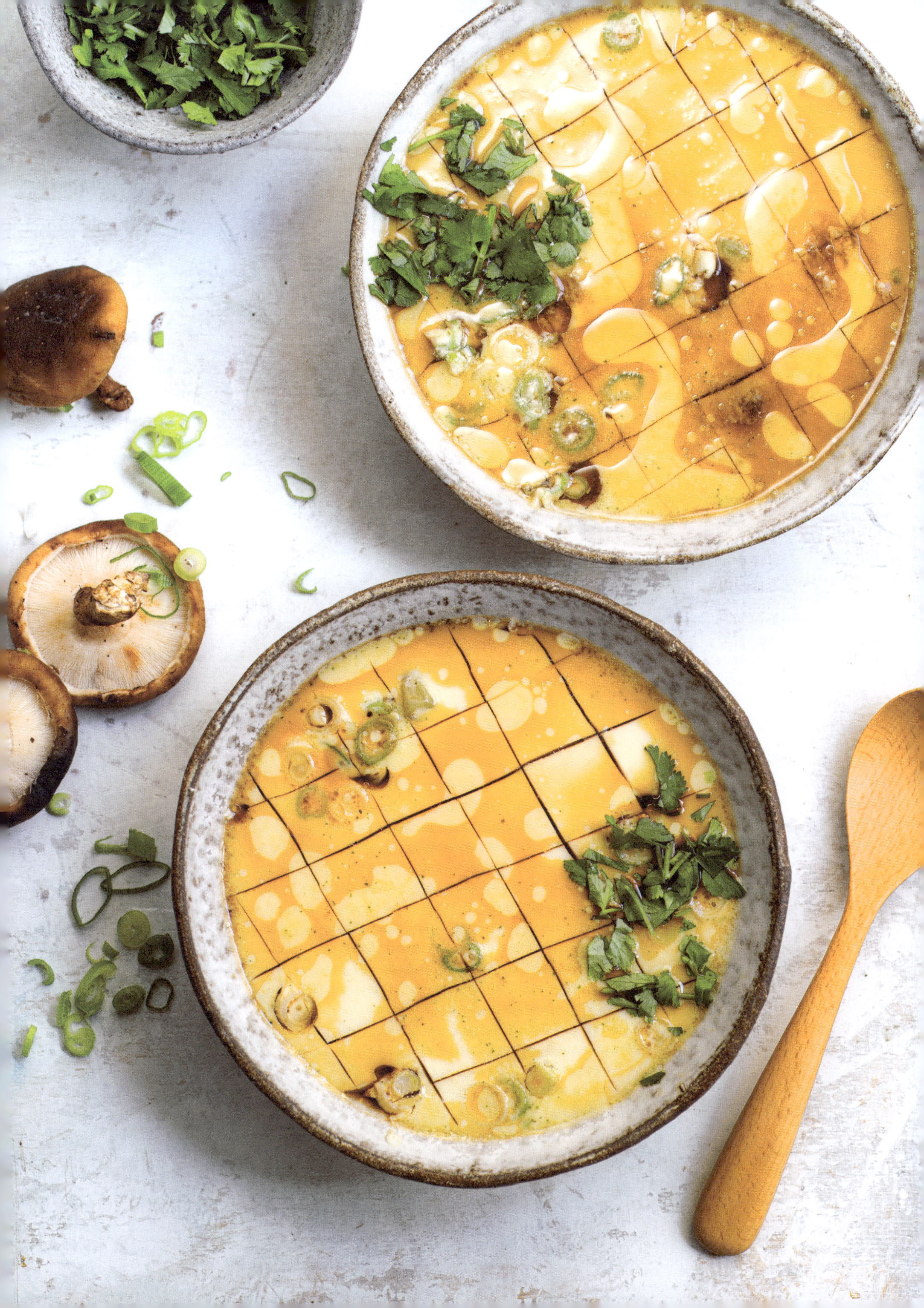

To boost production

Nut, Seed and Goji Berry Cereal Bars

MAKES **12 BARS** • PREPARATION TIME: **15 MINUTES** • COOKING TIME: **15 MINUTES**

75 g (3 oz) nuts of your choice (we have used 60 g/ 2¼ oz pecan nuts + 20 g/ ¾ oz hazelnuts)
50 g (2 oz) goji berries (or other dried fruits of your choice, such as apricots, dates, figs etc.)
70 g (2¾ oz) porridge oats
60 g (2¼ oz) seeds of your choice (we used 40 g/ 1½ oz flaxseeds + 20 g/ ¾ oz pumpkin seeds)
45 g (1¾ oz) coconut oil or butter
75 g (3 oz) agave syrup or honey

1. Preheat the oven to 180°C (350°F), Gas Mark 4.
2. Roughly chop the nuts and goji berries.
3. In a small blender, grind the oats and seeds, then transfer to a large bowl with the nuts and berries.
4. In a small saucepan, melt the coconut oil (or butter) with the agave syrup (or honey) over a low heat.
5. Pour the wet ingredients into the dry and combine thoroughly.
6. Spread the mixture into rectangular silicone cereal bar moulds, pressing down firmly.
7. Bake in the oven for 15 minutes.
8. Leave to cool completely before removing from the moulds.

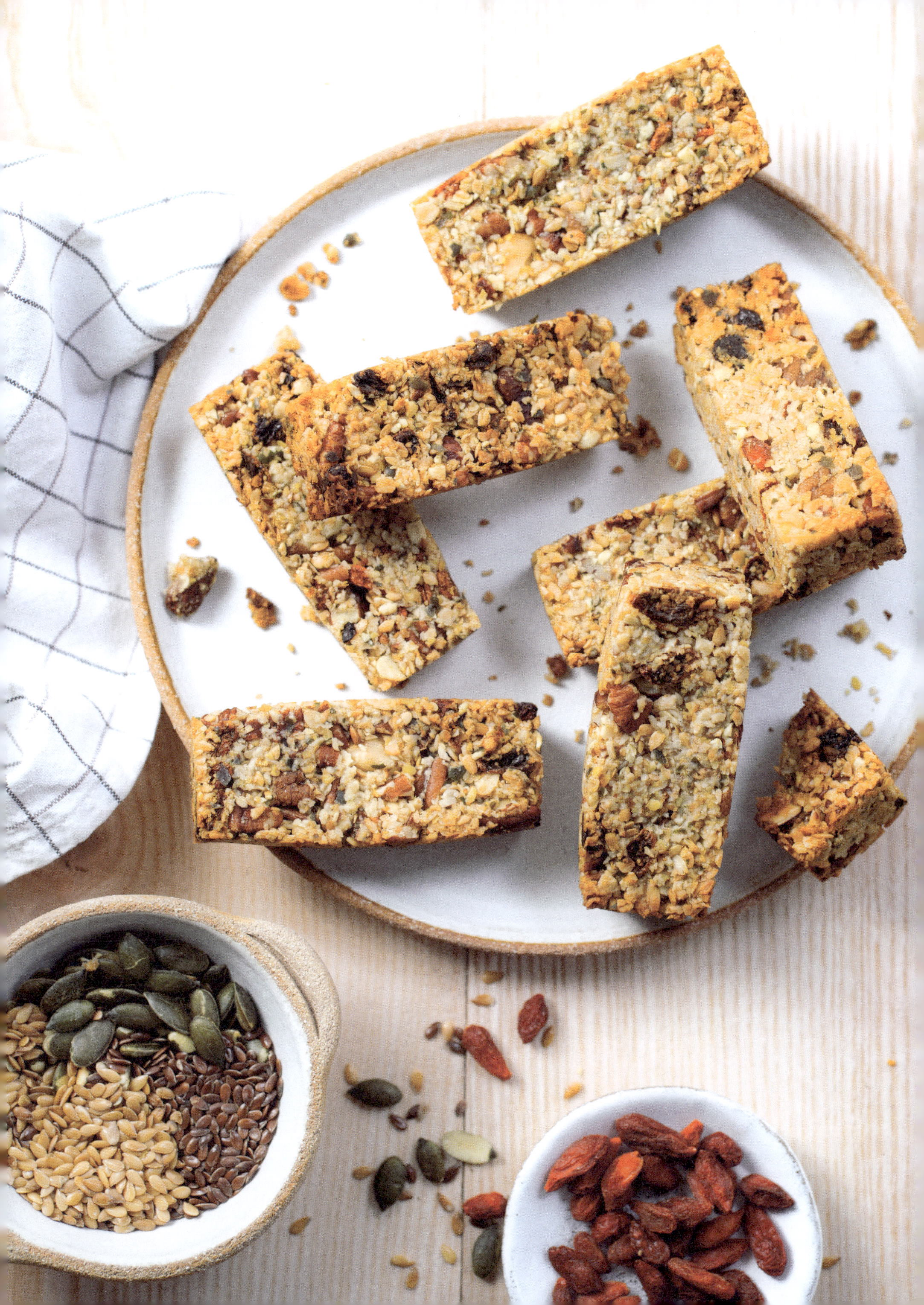

Seasonal Tips

Combine these foods with fruits and vegetables high in water content, for better hydration.

Include a lot of raw vegetables and smoothies in your diet to keep the nutrients intact and maximize their absorption.

Drink green iced tea and eat tomatoes marinated in olive oil to reinforce natural sun protection.

Drink water infused with citrus fruit and berries for refreshing and antioxidant-rich hydration.

Summer Recipes

Blueberry and Spirulina Smoothie Bowl

As a supplement

To boost production

SERVES **1** • PREPARATION TIME: **10 MINUTES**
RESTING TIME: MINIMUM **2 HOURS**

1 banana
135 g (4½ oz) frozen blueberries
1 teaspoon blue spirulina powder
250 ml (8 fl oz) coconut milk
2 teaspoons coconut cream
1 teaspoon green spirulina powder, plus extra to garnish
1 teaspoon coconut flakes
100 g (3½ oz) mixed dark berry fruits

1. The evening before (or at least 2 hours in advance), slice the banana and place in the freezer.
2. When ready to serve, blend the blueberries, frozen banana pieces, blue spirulina and coconut milk in a blender until smooth.
3. Mix the coconut cream with the green spirulina powder.
4. Spoon the smoothie into a bowl and top with the spirulina cream, coconut flakes, dark berries and a sprinkle of green spirulina powder over the top.

Tip

You can enrich your bowls with interesting fruits and seeds for collagen production, such as goji berries and hemp seeds.

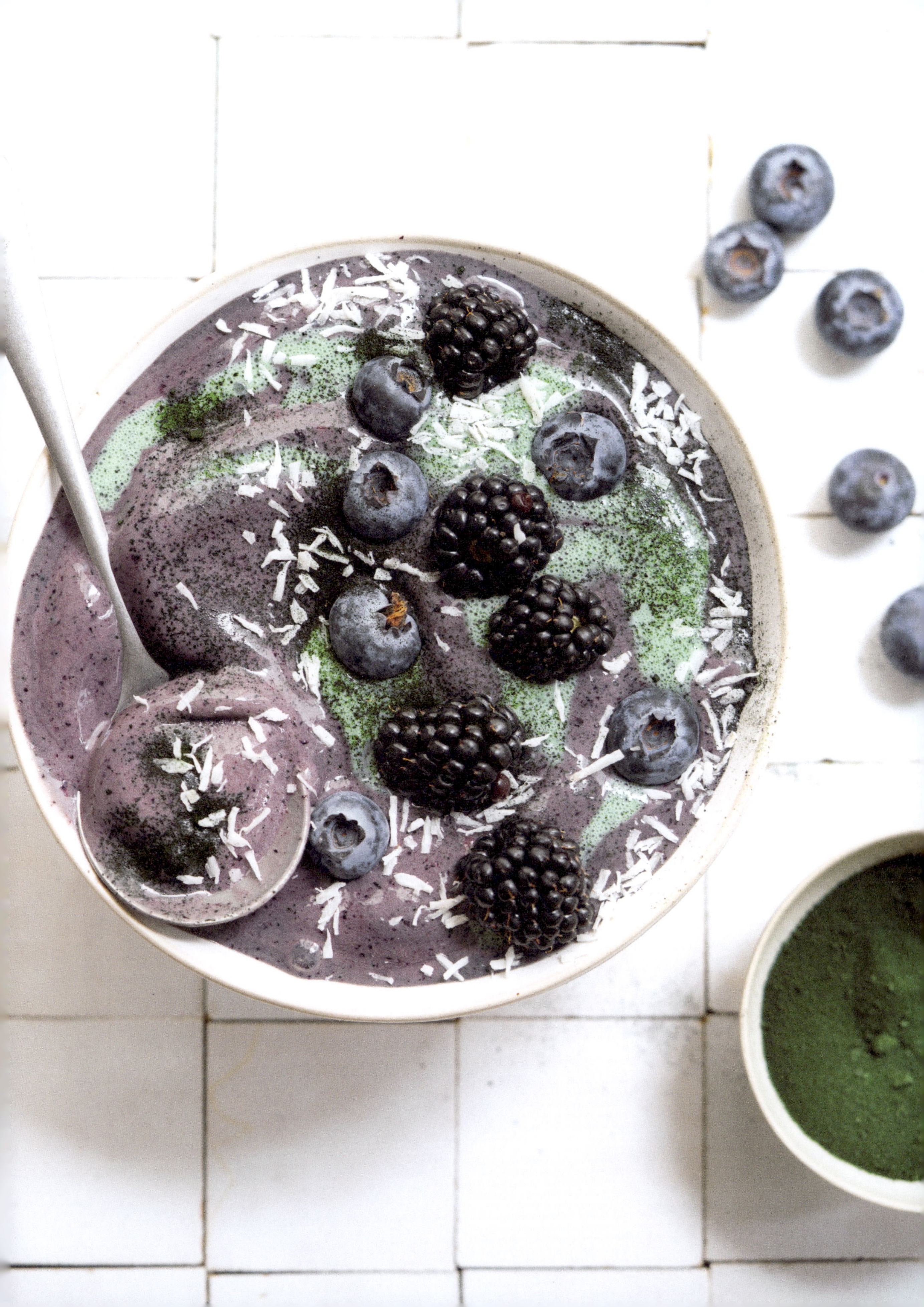

Pulled Pork Carnitas

SERVES **2** • PREPARATION TIME: **20 MINUTES** • COOKING TIME: **20 MINUTES**

6 small corn tortillas

FOR THE CITRUS-FLAVOURED PULLED PORK

200 g (7 oz) Pulled Pork (see page 94) or shredded meat from the Pork Stock (see page 19)
zest of ½ orange
100 ml (3½ fl oz) freshly squeezed orange juice (from about 1 orange)
3 tablespoons cider vinegar

FOR THE SALSA

½ red onion, finely diced
1 tomato, finely diced
200 g (7 oz) fresh pineapple, finely diced
½ avocado, finely diced
1 small red chilli, finely diced (optional)
juice of 1 lime
5 coriander sprigs, finely chopped

FOR THE CHIPOTLE SAUCE

50 g (2 oz) mayonnaise
100 g (3½ oz) crème fraîche
2 tablespoons lime juice
2 tablespoons chipotle sauce (or Sriracha sauce)

1. Reheat the Pulled Pork in a small saucepan. Add the orange zest, orange juice and vinegar and warm over a low heat for 15 minutes.
2. To make the salsa, mix all the ingredients together in a bowl.
3. To make the chipotle sauce, mix all the ingredients together in a separate bowl.
4. Warm the tortillas in a dry frying pan, then fill with the sauce, meat and salsa. Serve immediately.

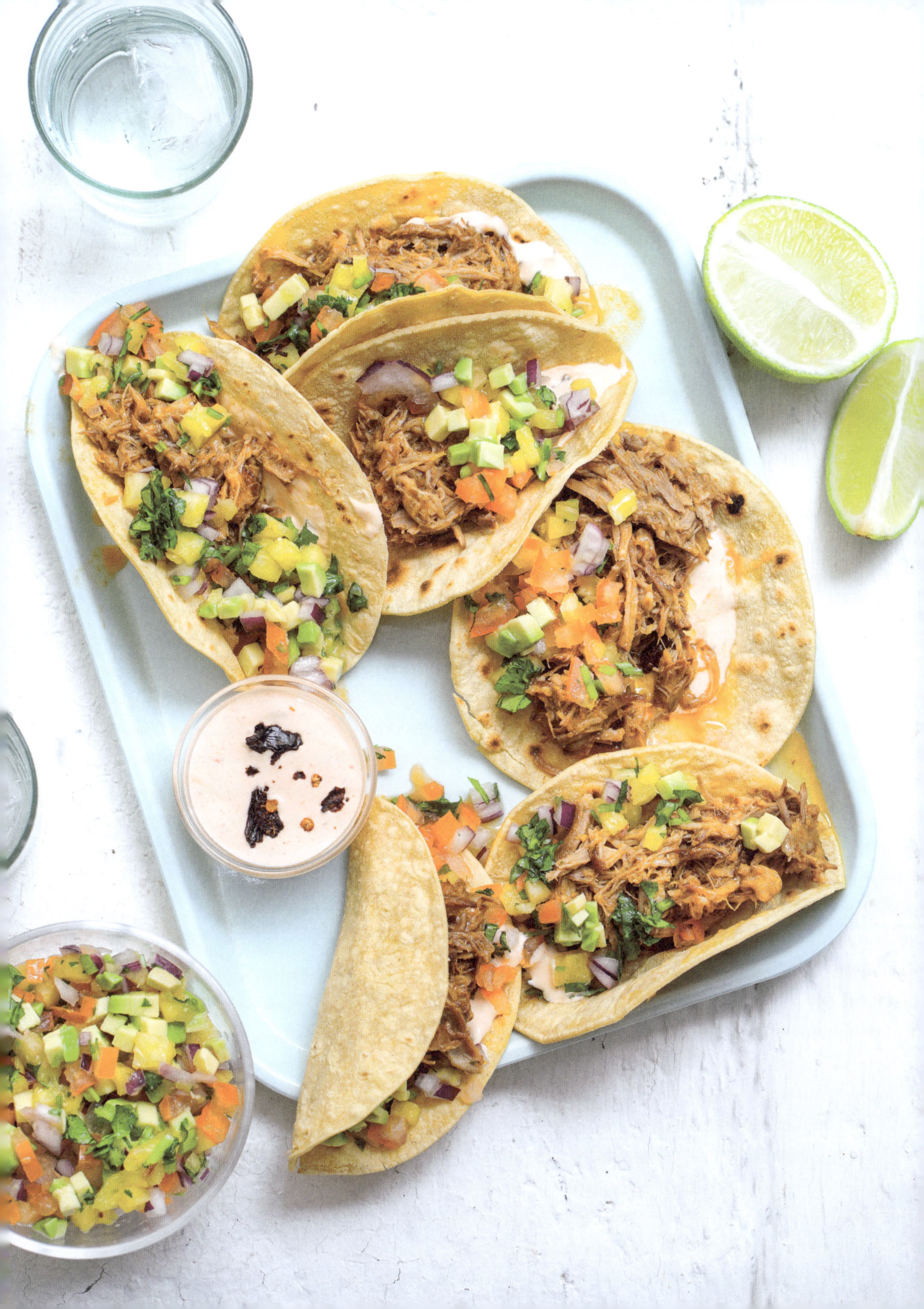

As a supplement

To boost production

Spiced Lamb Pittas

SERVES **2** • PREPARATION TIME: **10 MINUTES** • COOKING TIME: **30 MINUTES**

FOR THE SPICED LAMB

200 g (7 oz) braised lamb from the 7-Hour Lamb recipe (see page 34) (or use other leftover roast lamb)

½ teaspoon ground cumin

2 tablespoons olive oil (not needed if using 7-Hour Lamb)

TO SERVE

2 teaspoons za'atar

3 tablespoons olive oil

pinch of sea salt flakes

4 large wholegrain pitta breads

200 g (7 oz) labneh (or 100 g/3½ oz fromage frais and 100 g/3½ oz Greek-style yogurt)

50 g (2 oz) red cabbage, grated

100 g (3 ½ oz) carrot, grated

leaves from 4 mint sprigs

juice of 1 lemon

seeds from ½ pomegranate

1. Preheat the oven to 200°C (400°F), Gas Mark 6.
2. If using the 7-Hour Lamb, fry in a small amount of its cooking juice for about 15 minutes along with the cumin. If using other leftover lamb, toss the lamb in the olive oil, then grill for 5 minutes on each side for a medium finish.
3. Mix the za'atar with the olive oil and salt, then spread the mixture over each pitta bread.
4. Top each pitta with the labneh, grated cabbage and carrot, mint leaves and then the lamb. Add a squeeze of lemon juice and a sprinkle of pomegranate seeds before serving.

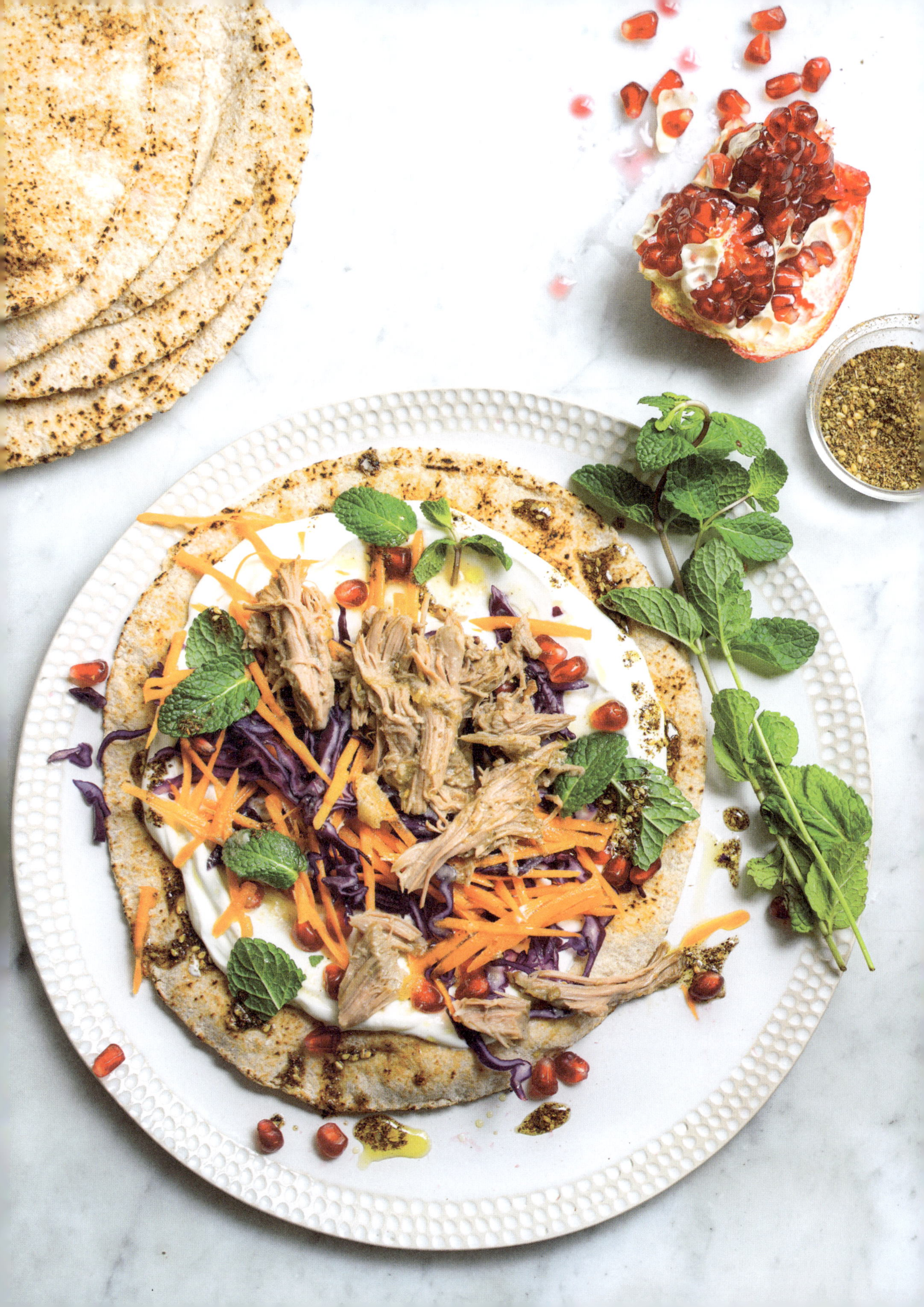

To boost production

Beef Tartare

SERVES **2** • PREPARATION TIME: **15 MINUTES**

250 g (8 oz) very fresh rump steak
15 g (½ oz) small capers, finely chopped
6 chives, finely chopped, plus extra to garnish
4 parsley sprigs, finely chopped
½ shallot, finely chopped
1 anchovy, finely chopped
4 gherkins, finely chopped

FOR THE SEASONING

2 tablespoons tomato ketchup
2 teaspoons Dijon mustard
1 teaspoon Worcestershire sauce
a few drops of Tabasco sauce (optional)
1 tablespoon olive oil
salt and pepper

TO SERVE

2 raw egg yolks
1 tablespoon caper berries (optional)
4 cherry tomatoes, quartered
a few salad leaves of your choice
mustard vinaigrette (optional)

1. Finely dice the steak with a sharp knife, then mix together with the chopped capers, chives, parsley, shallot, anchovy and gherkins in a large bowl.
2. Add the seasoning ingredients and mix again.
3. Shape the tartares by pressing the meat lightly into round pastry cutters placed on each serving plate, then remove the cutter.
4. Gently make a hollow in the top of each tartare and drop in the egg yolks without breaking them. Garnish with caper berries (if using), cherry tomatoes, chives, a few salad leaves and a mustard vinaigrette (if liked).

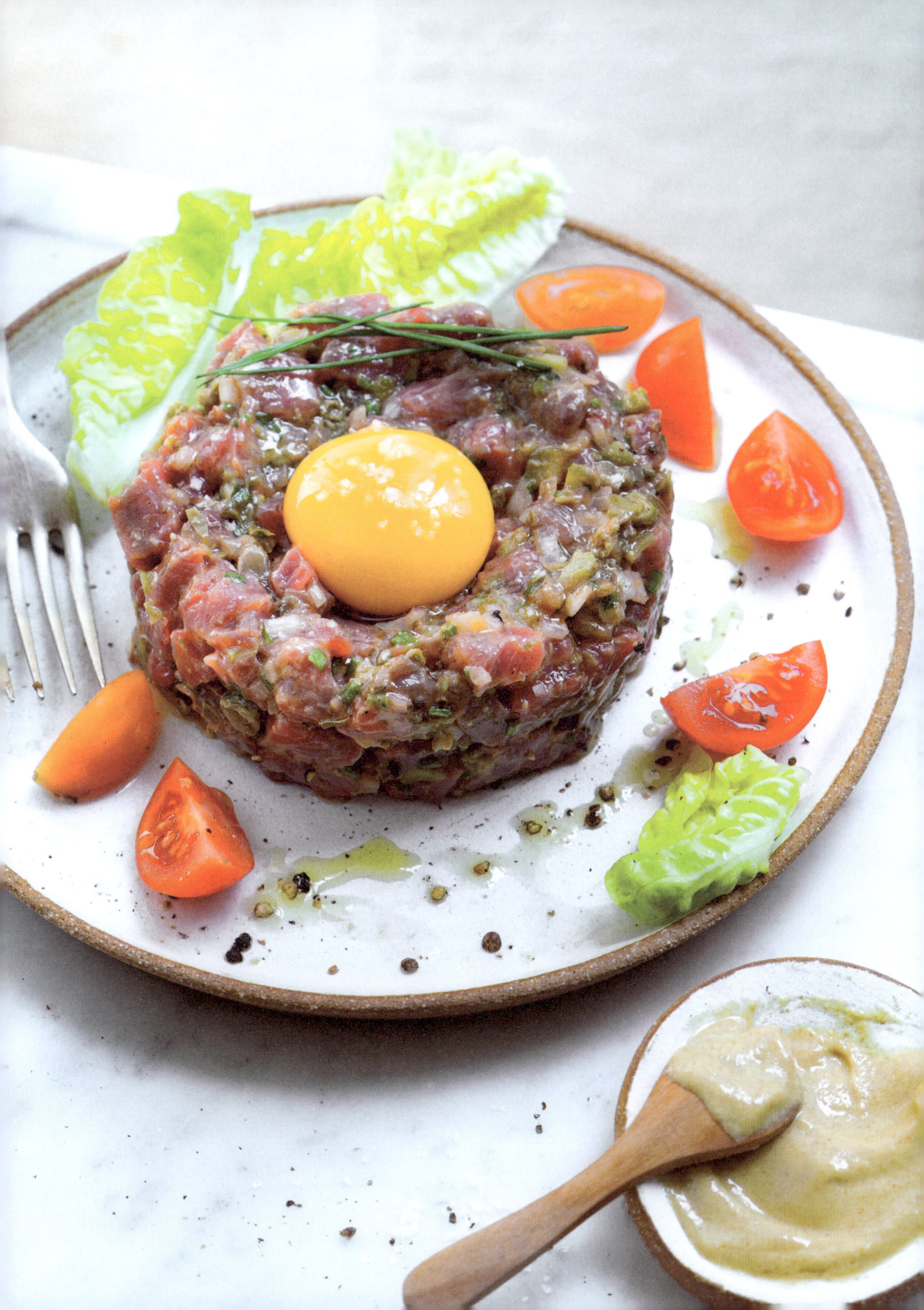

Braised Beef Pappardelle with Nettle Pesto

As a supplement

To boost production

SERVES **2** • PREPARATION TIME: **20 MINUTES** • COOKING TIME: **30 MINUTES**

250 g (8 oz) fresh pappardelle pasta
salt
a few parsley sprigs, to garnish

FOR THE BEEF RAGU

2 tablespoons olive oil
½ onion, finely chopped
2 garlic cloves, finely chopped
200 g (7 oz) braised beef from the French-style 'Pot-au-Feu' Broth (see page 17), shredded
4 thyme sprigs, finely chopped
400 ml (14 fl oz) French-style 'Pot-au-Feu' Broth (see page 17)

FOR THE NETTLE PESTO

50 g (2 oz) fresh nettle leaves (foraged or try your greengrocer)
50 g (2 oz) almonds (or pine nuts)
1 tablespoon white vinegar
80 g (3 oz) Parmesan cheese, grated
50 ml (2 fl oz) olive oil
50 ml (2 fl oz) sunflower oil
1 garlic clove
1 teaspoon malted yeast
salt and pepper

1. Heat the oil in a large saucepan. When hot, sauté the onion and garlic for 3 minutes, then add the shredded beef, thyme and broth. Reheat over a low heat for 15 minutes without covering, so that the broth can reduce down and the flavours become more concentrated.
2. To make the pesto, place the nettle leaves in a saucepan of salted boiling water and cook for 3 minutes before transferring them to a large bowl of cold water.
3. Drain the nettles and add to a food processor along with the remaining pesto ingredients. Blitz until you have a smooth, creamy paste.
4. Bring a large pan of salted water to the boil. Add the pappardelle and cook according to the packet instructions, then drain.
5. Tip the pappardelle into the saucepan with the beef and incorporate the pesto. Combine everything thoroughly before serving, garnished with a few parsley sprigs.

Tip

Pesto is traditionally made with pine nuts, but you can use any nuts of your choice.

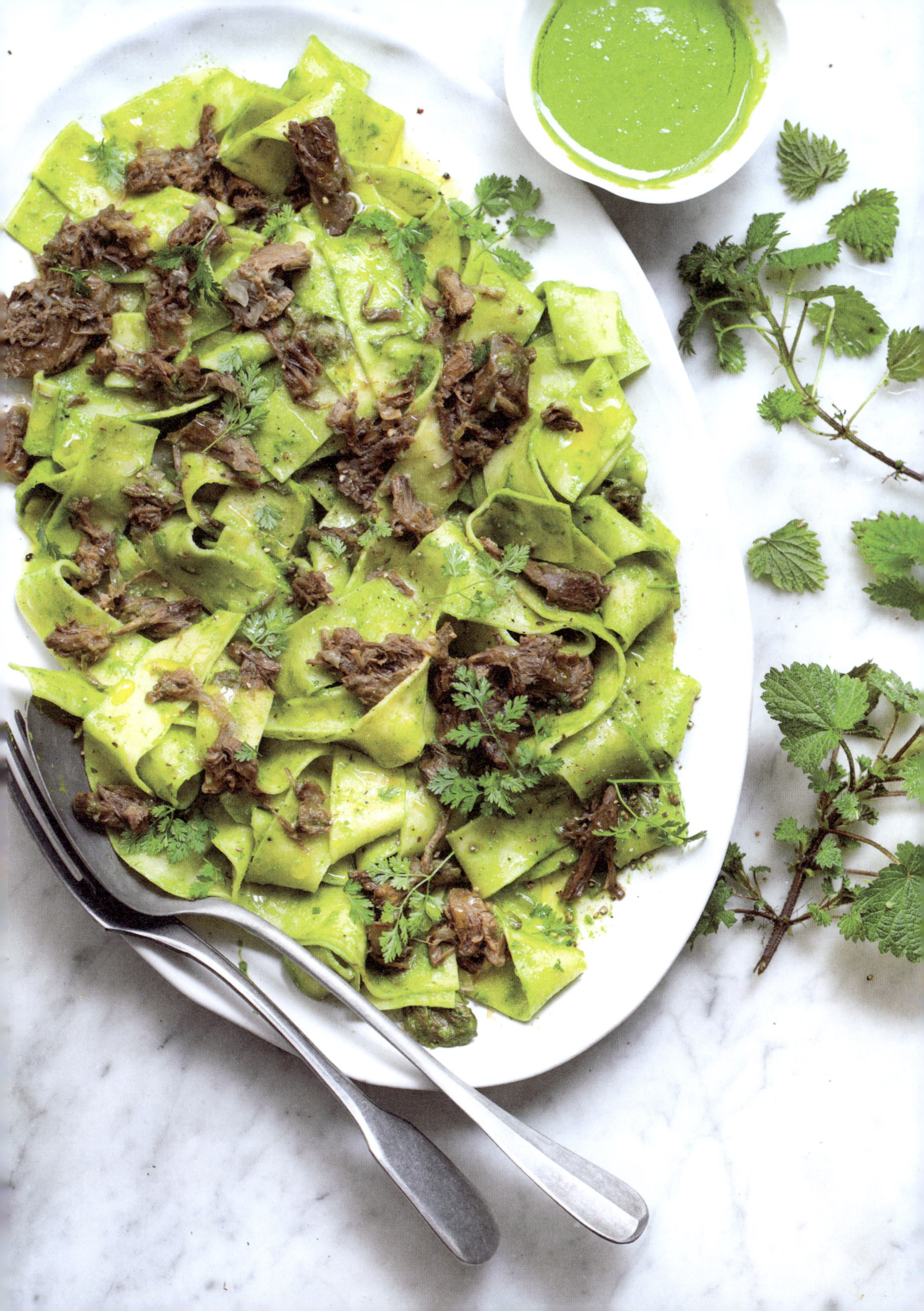

As a supplement

To boost production

Hake Steaks with Red Rice

SERVES **2** • PREPARATION TIME: **15 MINUTES** • COOKING TIME: **30 MINUTES**

500 ml (17 fl oz) Fish Stock (see page 20)
250 g (8 oz) mix of julienned vegetables (carrots, celeriac, leek etc.)
2 hake steaks
100 g (3½ oz) frozen broad beans or peas
2 tablespoons cornflour
2 tablespoons cold water
2 tablespoons double cream
1 bunch of dill, finely chopped
salt and pepper

FOR THE HERBY RED RICE

100 g (3½ oz) red rice
a bunch of aromatic herbs of your choice (chervil, basil, coriander, tarragon etc.), finely chopped
100 g (3½ oz) broccoli, finely chopped
1 tablespoon flaxseed oil
salt and pepper

1. Cook the red rice according to the packet instructions (usually about 30 minutes).
2. Meanwhile, bring the Fish Stock to the boil in a large saucepan. Add the vegetable mix and cook for 10 minutes.
3. Add the hake steaks and frozen broad beans to the pan and cook for a further 5 minutes.
4. Using a slotted spoon, remove the vegetables and fish and set aside.
5. Mix the cornflour with the cold water and add to the saucepan along with the cream, dill (reserving a little for garnish) and some salt and pepper. Stir and gently simmer for 5 minutes.
6. Drain the rice and mix in the aromatic herbs, broccoli, flaxseed oil and a little salt and pepper.
7. Serve the fish and vegetables with the sauce, garnished with the reserved dill, with the rice on the side.

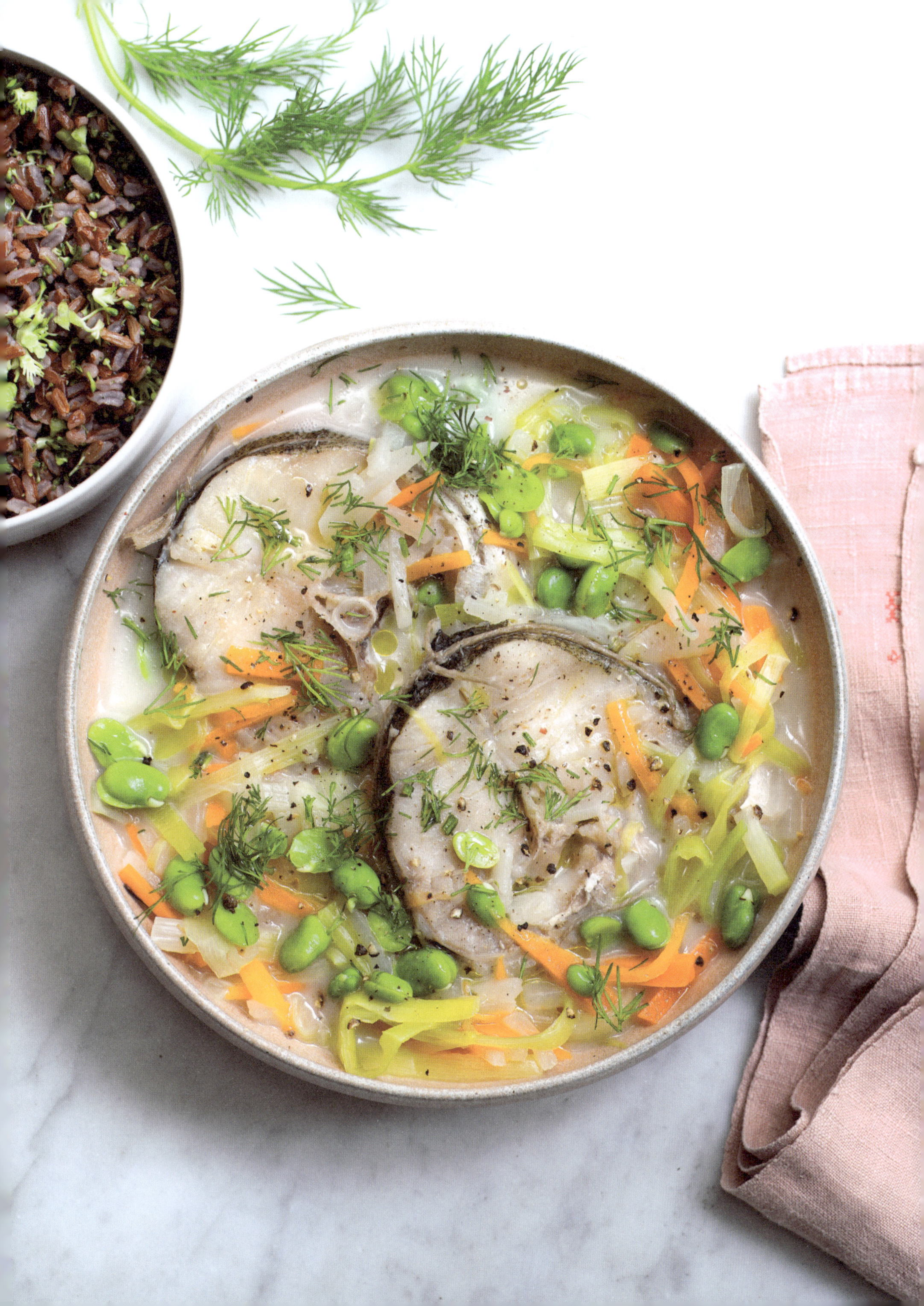

COLLAGEN THERAPY • SUMMER

Protection and hydration for the skin

Summer pushes the skin to its limits with sun exposure and environmental damage. This treatment focuses on protecting the skin, cell renewal and hydration. Antioxidants, fatty acids and marine collagen are key to keeping skin firm, elastic and UV resistant.

AIM

To protect the skin from UV rays, prevent skin ageing and maintain hydration.

To boost production

KEY NUTRIENTS

To stimulate collagen production naturally, some essential cofactors are required.

- **Vitamin C** (citrus fruit, red berries, peppers, parsley and broccoli)
- **Zinc and copper** (oysters, seeds, dark chocolate, cashew nuts, sunflower seeds, lean red meat)
- **Omega-3 fatty acids** (oily fish, avocado, flaxseed)
- **Antioxidants** (green tea, berries, raw cacao, carrots, turmeric)

Things To Know

- **For natural UV protection:** tomatoes, carrots, sweet potatoes, red peppers, apricots, mangoes
- **For hydration and skin elasticity:** watermelon, melon, cucumber, celery, lettuce, coconut water

As a supplement

KEY FOODS

The following foods contain bioavailable collagen to maintain plump and elastic skin despite exposure to the sun.

Fish, including the skin and bones (salmon, sardines, mackerel)

Chicken (skin and cartilage)

Bone broth (beef, chicken, fish)

Egg white (rich in proline, a precursor to collagen)

Pork rind (baked, jellied, in homemade pâté)

Natural gelatine and collagen powder

	DAY 1	DAY 2
BREAKFAST	**Blueberry and Spirulina** Smoothie Bowl • see page 64 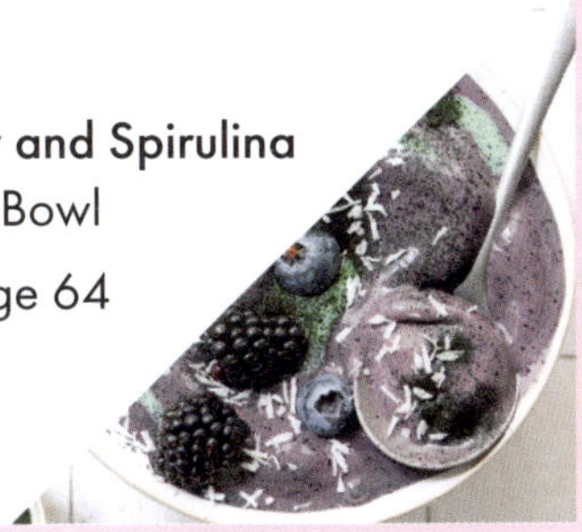	**Marine collagen smoothie: blend together coconut water, powdered marine collagen, kiwi fruit and almond milk**
LUNCH	**Fresh salad:** combine a small amount of chicken, cucumber, rocket leaves, sunflower seeds, cherry tomatoes and olive oil	**Tuna tartare with mango and fresh herbs:** dice some fresh tuna, slice the mango and chop the herbs, mix together and season with a drizzle of lime juice and olive oil
SNACK	**Homemade Kombucha with Red Berries** • see page 25 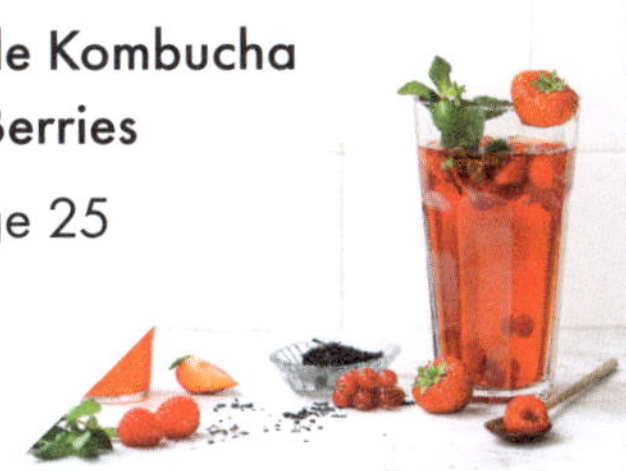	**Raspberry-Matcha Tiramisu** • see page 88 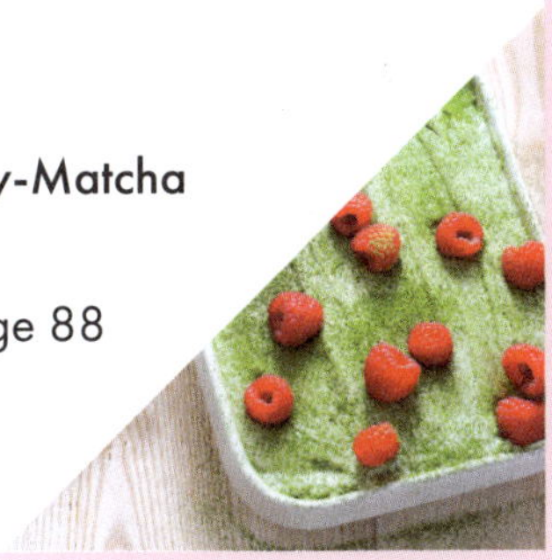
DINNER	**Chirashi Bowl** • see page 78 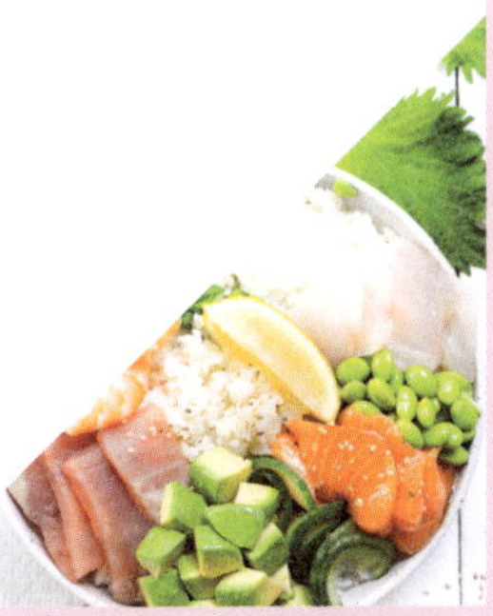	**Fish Stock** • see page 20 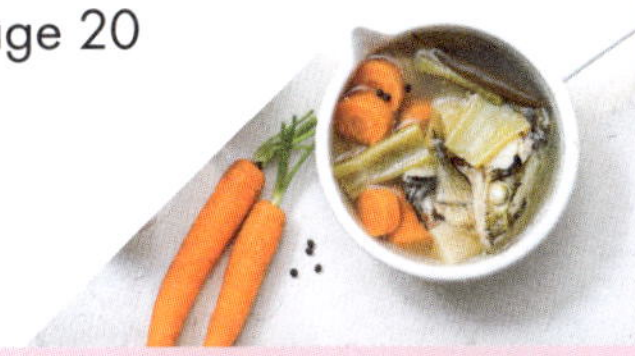

Chirashi Bowl

As a supplement

To boost production

SERVES **2** • PREPARATION TIME: **30 MINUTES** • COOKING TIME: **15 MINUTES**
RESTING TIME: **10 MINUTES**

FOR THE VINEGARED RICE

200 g (7 oz) sushi rice
400 ml (14 fl oz) water
2 teaspoons caster sugar
50 g (2 oz) rice vinegar
½ teaspoon salt

TO SERVE

150 g (5 oz) edamame beans
1 boneless salmon steak
1 tuna steak
1 boneless, skinless sea bream or sea bass fillet
8 cooked shelled prawns, deveined
1 avocado, pitted, peeled and diced
100 g (3½ oz) cucumber, thinly sliced
4 shiso leaves (optional)
2 teaspoons fish roe
½ lemon, halved

1. Rinse the rice three times, then drain well and place in a rice cooker or saucepan. Add the measured water, cover and bring to the boil. As soon as it starts to boil, reduce the heat and simmer for 12 minutes with the lid on. Turn off the heat and leave to steam for 10 minutes, keeping the lid on.
2. Place the sugar, vinegar and salt in a saucepan. Heat until the salt and sugar are dissolved, then pour over the warm rice. Carefully fold through using a large, flat spoon.
3. Cook the edamame beans for 5 minutes in a saucepan of boiling water, then chill in a bowl of cold water.
4. Cut the fish into thick slices.
5. Divide the cooled rice between 2 bowls and garnish with the fish, prawns, edamame beans, avocado, cucumber, shiso leaves (if using) and fish roe. Serve each with a lemon wedge for squeezing.

Tip

You could also serve with a small amount of wasabi, pickled ginger and soy sauce.

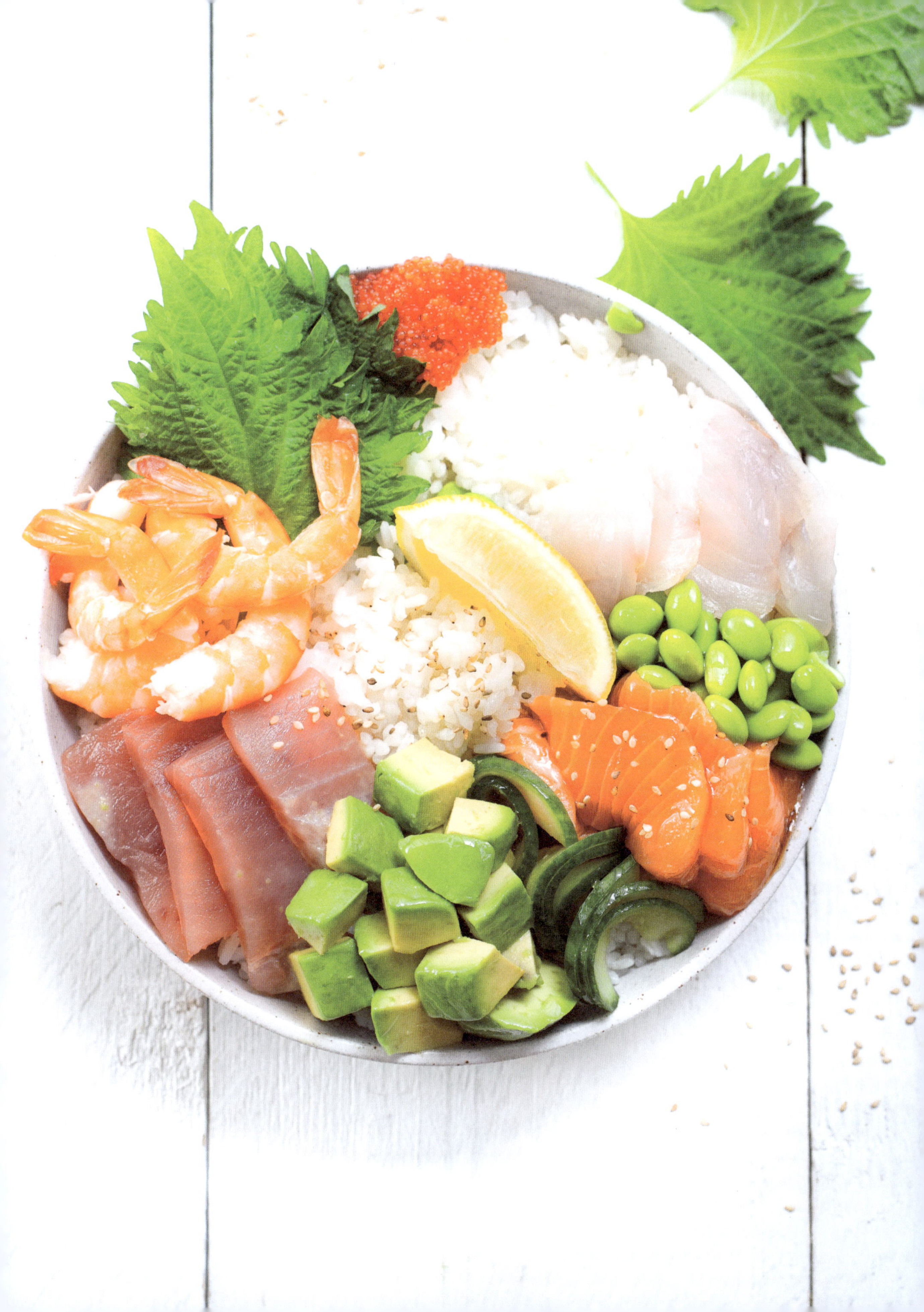

Bulgur Wheat, Goats' Cheese and Pistachio Tabbouleh

To **boost** production

SERVES **2** • PREPARATION TIME: **25 MINUTES** • COOKING TIME: **10 MINUTES**

FOR THE TABBOULEH

80 g (3 oz) bulgur wheat
1 bunch of parsley, finely chopped
5 mint sprigs, finely chopped
½ red onion, finely chopped
seeds of ½ pomegranate
1 grapefruit, peeled and segmented
juice of 1 lemon
2 teaspoons za'atar
2 tablespoons olive oil
salt and pepper

FOR THE PISTACHIO GOATS' CHEESE

200 g (7 oz) fresh goats' cheese
30 g (1¼ oz) pistachios
salt and pepper

1. Cook the bulgur wheat according to the packet instructions. Drain and leave to cool.
2. Mix all the tabbouleh ingredients in a large salad bowl. Season with salt and pepper and store in the refrigerator until ready to serve.
3. In a bowl, mix the fresh goats' cheese with a little salt and pepper, then divide into 12 portions and shape into balls.
4. In a food processor, pulse the pistachios until you have a coarse powder, then place in a bowl. Roll the goats' cheese balls in the ground pistachios and serve with the tabbouleh.

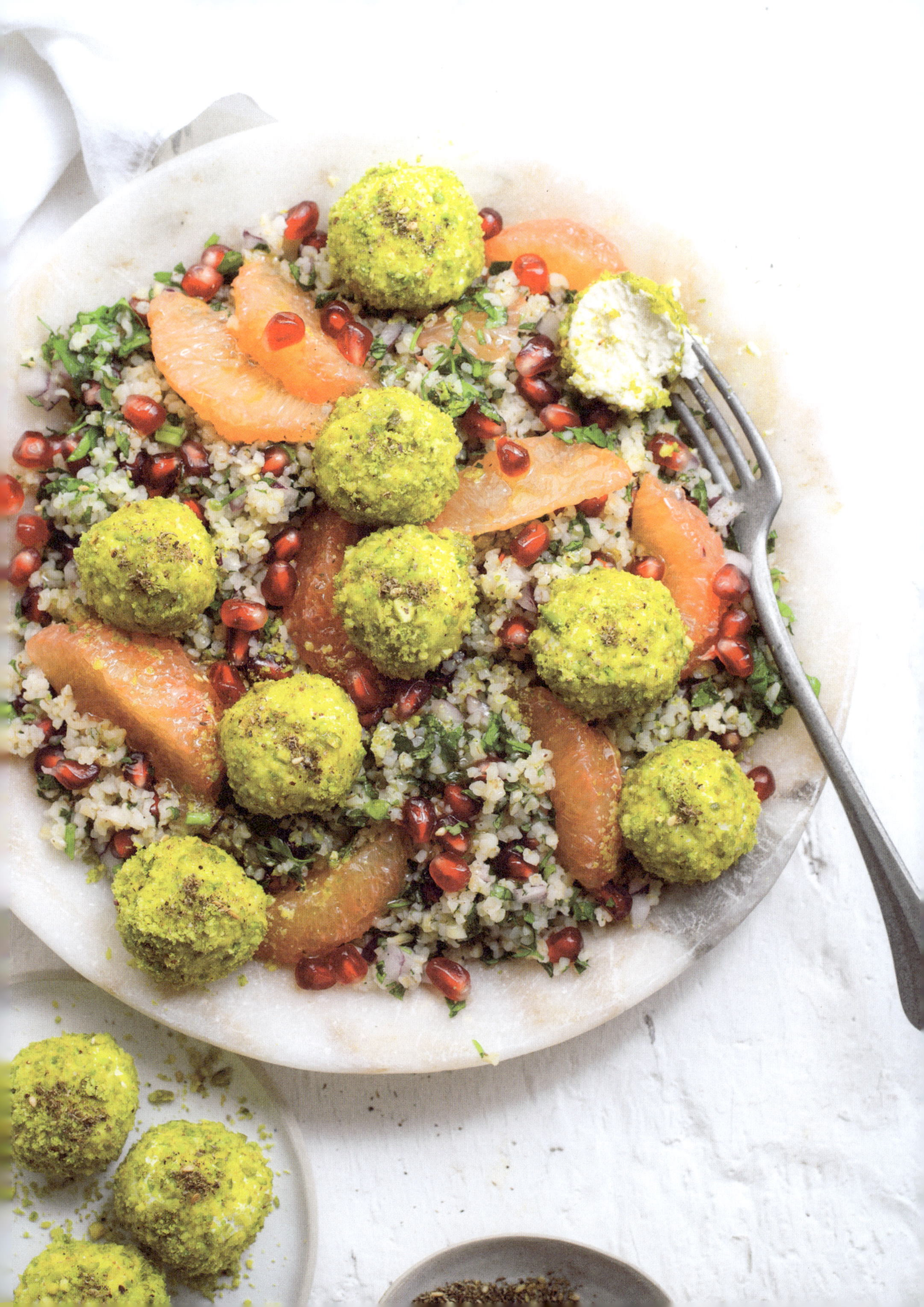

To boost production

Shakshuka with Garlic Toasts

SERVES **2** • PREPARATION TIME: **25 MINUTES** • COOKING TIME: **40–45 MINUTES**

1 tablespoon olive oil
1 onion, finely sliced
1 garlic clove, finely chopped
½ teaspoon ground cumin
small pinch of smoked paprika
2 red peppers, deseeded and cut into strips
400 g (13 oz) tomatoes, coarsely grated
2 eggs
60 g (2¼ oz) feta cheese
salt and pepper
parsley leaves, to garnish

FOR THE GARLIC TOASTS

2 tablespoons olive oil
4 slices of rustic bread
1 garlic clove, peeled

1. Heat the oil in a large frying pan over a medium heat. Sauté the onion and garlic for about 3 minutes, then add the spices and some salt and pepper and cook for a further minute.
2. Stir the peppers into the pan, then cover and cook for 15–20 minutes until soft.
3. Add the tomatoes and cook uncovered for 15 minutes.
4. By now, the mixture should have reduced and the tomato liquid should have evaporated. Make 2 hollows in the stew using a large spoon. Break the eggs into the hollows, taking care not to break the yolks. Cover and cook for 5–6 minutes over a low heat, keeping a close eye, until the whites are cooked but the yolks remain runny.
5. Meanwhile, make the garlic toasts. Heat the oil in a separate frying pan and toast the slices of bread on both sides. Rub the surface of each toast with the garlic clove.
6. Crumble the feta over the top of the shakshuka and garnish with some parsley leaves. Serve immediately with the toasted breads on the side.

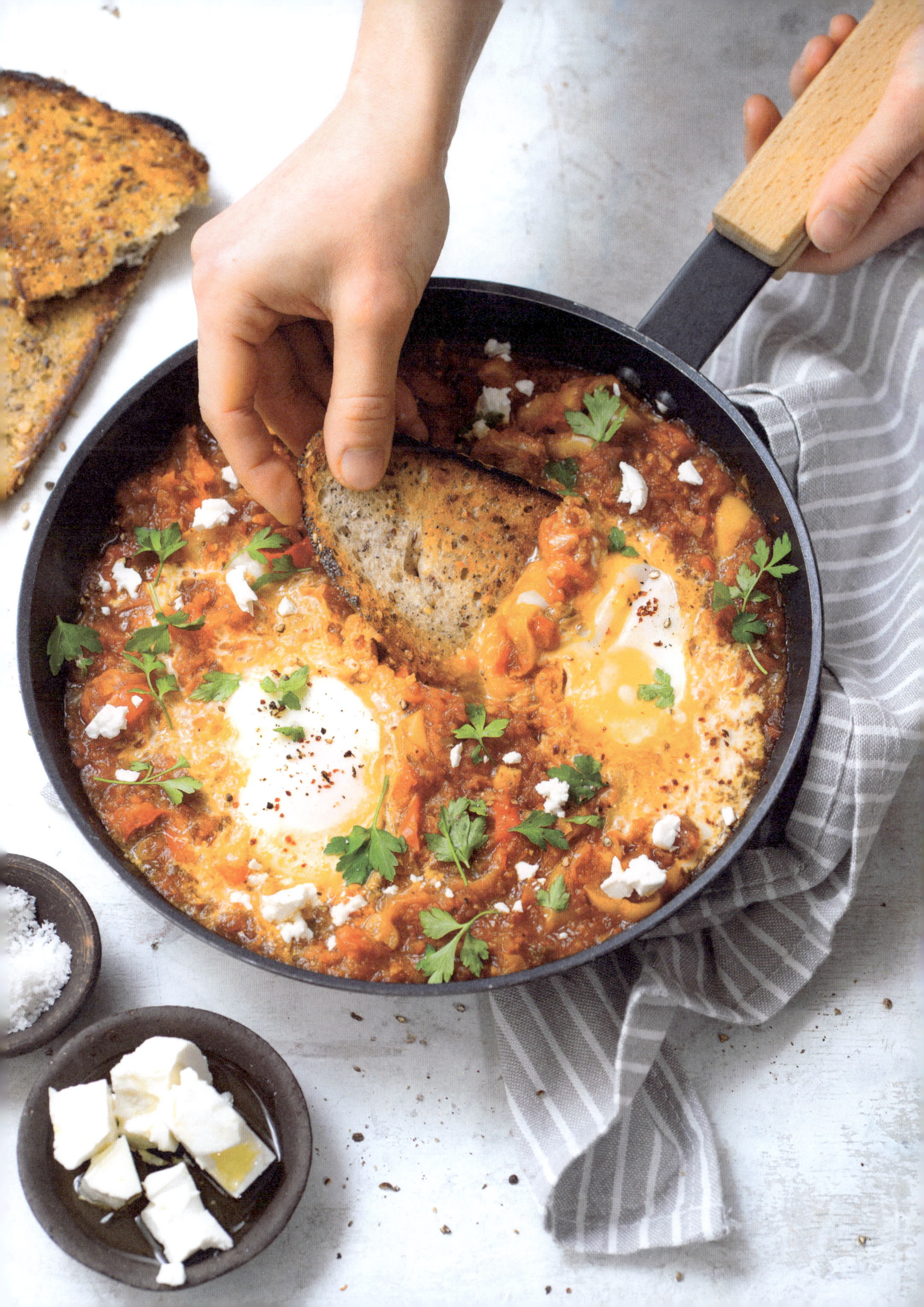

To boost production

Veggie Chilli

SERVES **2** • PREPARATION TIME: **10 MINUTES** • COOKING TIME: **35 MINUTES**

1 tablespoon olive oil
½ brown onion, finely chopped
1 garlic clove, finely chopped
1 teaspoon chilli powder
1 teaspoon ground cumin
1 teaspoon smoked paprika
1 teaspoon dried oregano
2 tomatoes, diced
1 yellow pepper, deseeded and diced
2 carrots, peeled and diced
200 ml (7 fl oz) Vegetable Stock (see page 23)
400 g (13 oz) can of crushed tomatoes
140 g (4½ oz) drained canned kidney beans
140 g (4½ oz) drained canned sweetcorn
100 g (3½ oz) tricolour quinoa
a few parsley or coriander sprigs
2 tablespoons Greek-style yogurt
lime wedges
salt and pepper

1. Heat the oil in a casserole dish. When hot, sauté the onion and garlic for 2 minutes, then add the spices, oregano, tomatoes, pepper and carrots. Cook for a further 5 minutes.
2. Pour in the Vegetable Stock and crushed tomatoes, and season with salt and pepper. Cover and simmer for 20 minutes.
3. Add the kidney beans and sweetcorn and cook for a further 5 minutes.
4. Meanwhile, cook the quinoa in a large saucepan of boiling water according to the packet instructions.
5. Serve the chilli and quinoa garnished with parsley or coriander sprigs, with a spoonful of Greek-style yogurt and a lime wedge for squeezing.

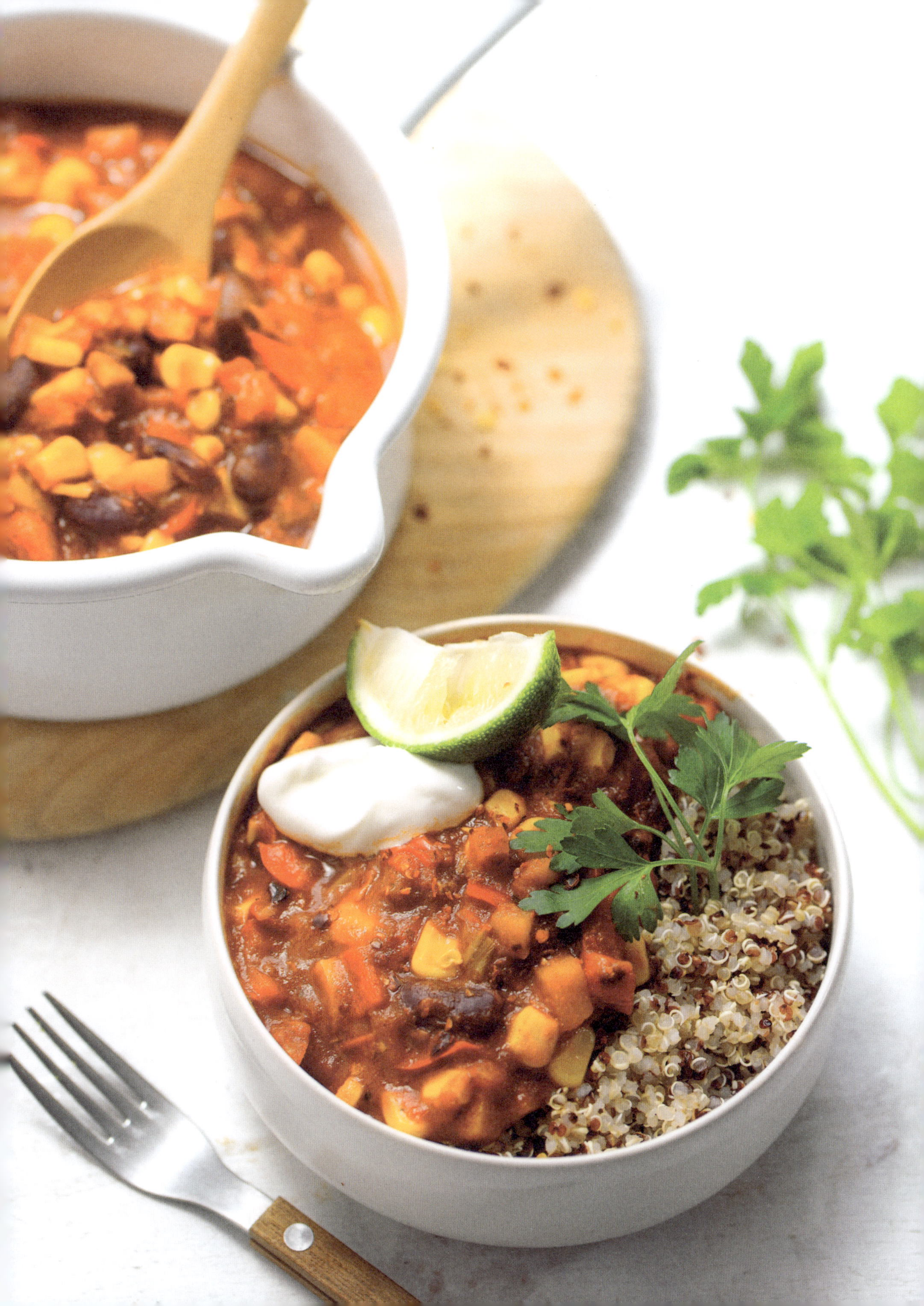

Poached Egg on Avocado Toast

SERVES **2** • PREPARATION TIME: **25 MINUTES** • COOKING TIME: **15 MINUTES**

4 large slices of seeded bread
2 tablespoons pumpkin seeds
chilli oil (or 1 tablespoon of Sriracha sauce)

FOR THE PICKLED RED ONIONS

½ red onion, thinly sliced
juice of 1 lime
1 teaspoon olive oil
salt and pepper

FOR THE POACHED EGGS

1 tablespoon white vinegar
4 eggs

FOR THE SPEEDY GUACAMOLE

1 avocado, pitted and peeled
juice of ½ lime
pinch of ground cumin
pinch of smoked paprika
5 coriander sprigs, chopped
1 tomato, chopped
salt and pepper

1. First, make the pickled onions. In a bowl, mix the red onion with the lime juice and olive oil. Season with salt and pepper. Set aside.
2. To make the poached eggs, bring a pan of water to the boil and add the white vinegar. Break 1 egg into a ramekin. Using a whisk, create a vortex in the middle of the water in the pan, then gently slide the egg into the vortex. Simmer for about 1 minute, then remove the poached egg from the water with a slotted spoon and place it in a bowl of cold water. Drain and place on kitchen paper. Repeat the process with the remaining 3 eggs.
3. For the speedy guacamole, mash the avocado flesh with the lime juice, cumin and paprika. Stir in the coriander and tomato and season with salt and pepper.
4. Toast the slices of bread, then spread each slice with the guacamole and top with pickled onions, a poached egg, some pumpkin seeds and a dash of chilli oil.

Tip

Non-vegetarians could also add a few slices of smoked trout.

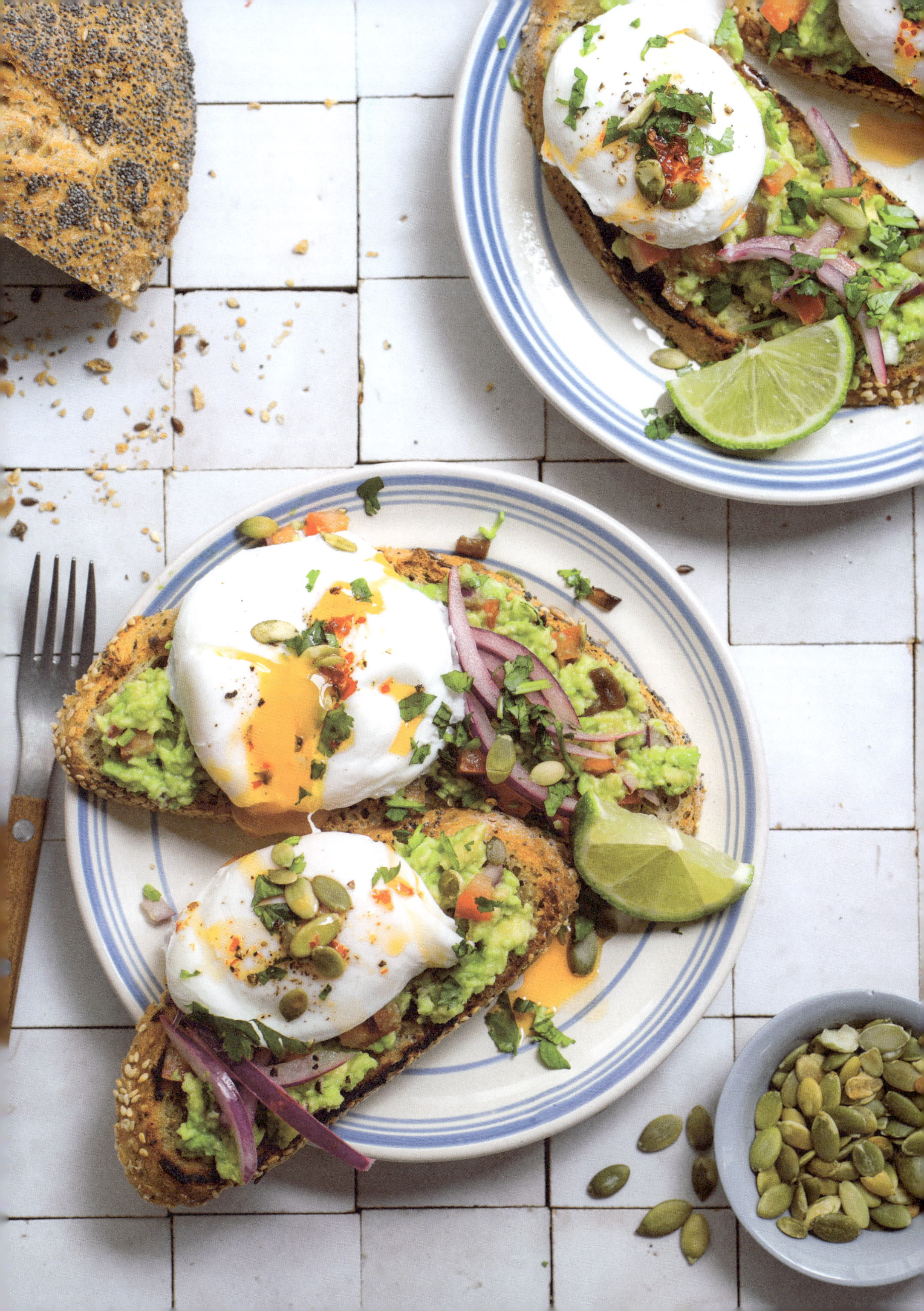

Raspberry Matcha Tiramisu

SERVES **6** • PREPARATION TIME: **25 MINUTES** • COOKING TIME: **5 MINUTES**
RESTING TIME: **2 HOURS**

200 ml (7 fl oz) hot water
2 tablespoons matcha tea, plus extra to decorate
20 sponge fingers
125 g (4 oz) fresh raspberries, to decorate

FOR THE MASCARPONE AND MATCHA CREAM

5 g (¼ oz) powdered gelatine (or 3 gelatine leaves)
1 teaspoon matcha tea
60 g (2¼ oz) caster sugar
1 egg plus 3 egg yolks
250 g (8 oz) mascarpone

1. First, make the mascarpone and matcha cream. Place the powdered gelatine (or gelatine leaves) in a small bowl of cold water to rehydrate. Leave to soak for about 5 minutes.
2. Melt the rehydrated gelatine powder (or the drained leaves) in the microwave, then sift the matcha tea over the gelatine and mix well.
3. In a large bowl with an electric mixer, beat the sugar, whole egg and egg yolks for 3 minutes at high speed until pale and frothy. Incorporate the matcha mixture while continuing to beat, this time at low speed.
4. In another bowl, beat the mascarpone until soft. Add the mascarpone to the matcha mixture while continuing to beat.
5. In a small bowl, combine the hot water (80°C/175°F maximum) with the matcha tea and mix well with a whisk.
6. Quickly dip half of the sponge fingers into the warm matcha tea, then lay them out along the bottom of a fairly deep rectangular dish (about 20cm/8 inches wide). Cover with half of the mascarpone and matcha cream. Repeat the process and smooth over the surface. Cover with cling film and chill for at least 2 hours in the refrigerator.
7. Sprinkle with matcha and decorate with raspberries just before serving.

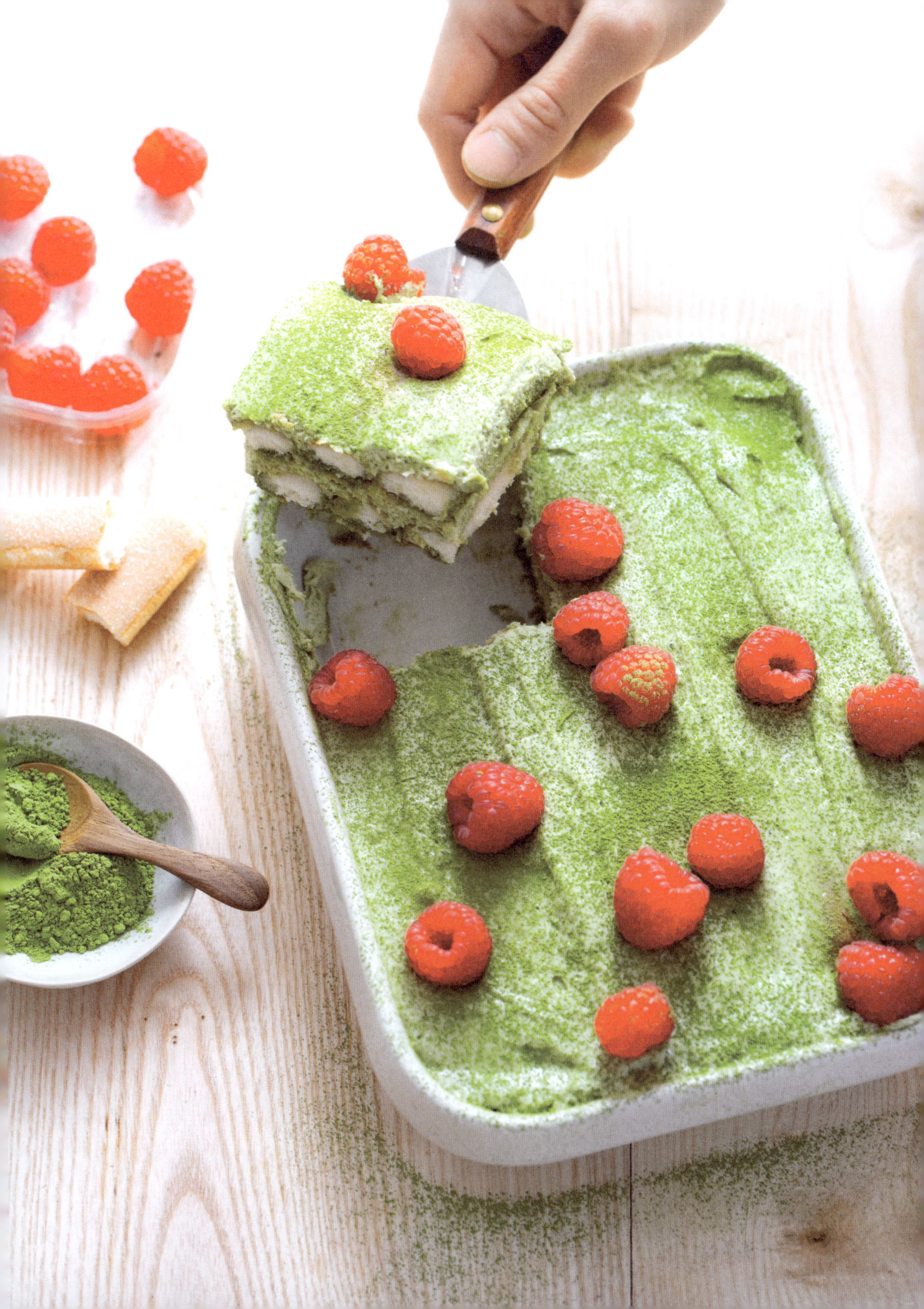

Seasonal Tips

Eat soups and stews to enhance the absorption of nutrients, while also getting the 'warming' benefits.

Combine collagen sources with vitamin C to maximize its absorption.

Include seeds and nuts in soups and salads for a boost of vital minerals.

Drink an infusion of turmeric and ginger in the evening to calm joint pain and encourage night-time regeneration.

Autumn Recipes

To boost production

Banana Pancakes

MAKES **10** PANCAKES • PREPARATION TIME: **5 MINUTES** • COOKING TIME: **10 MINUTES**

2 ripe bananas, peeled
2 eggs
1 tablespoon Skyr or Greek-style yogurt
40 g (1 ½ oz) ground almonds
60 g (2 ¼ oz) plain flour
pinch of bicarbonate of soda or baking powder
1 dose (see packet instructions for dosage) of collagen powder (optional)
1 teaspoon coconut oil

TO SERVE

handful of red berries
2 tablespoons Skyr or Greek-style yogurt
dash of lemon juice
1 tablespoon honey, or to taste

1. In a bowl, mash the bananas and mix with the eggs and yogurt.
2. In a separate bowl, mix together the ground almonds, flour and bicarbonate of soda or baking powder (and the collagen powder, if desired).
3. Add the dry mix to the banana mixture and combine thoroughly.
4. Heat the coconut oil in a frying pan. When hot, fry spoonfuls of the batter for 2 minutes on each side.
5. Serve with some red berries, a spoonful of yogurt, a squeeze of lemon juice and a generous drizzle of honey, to taste.

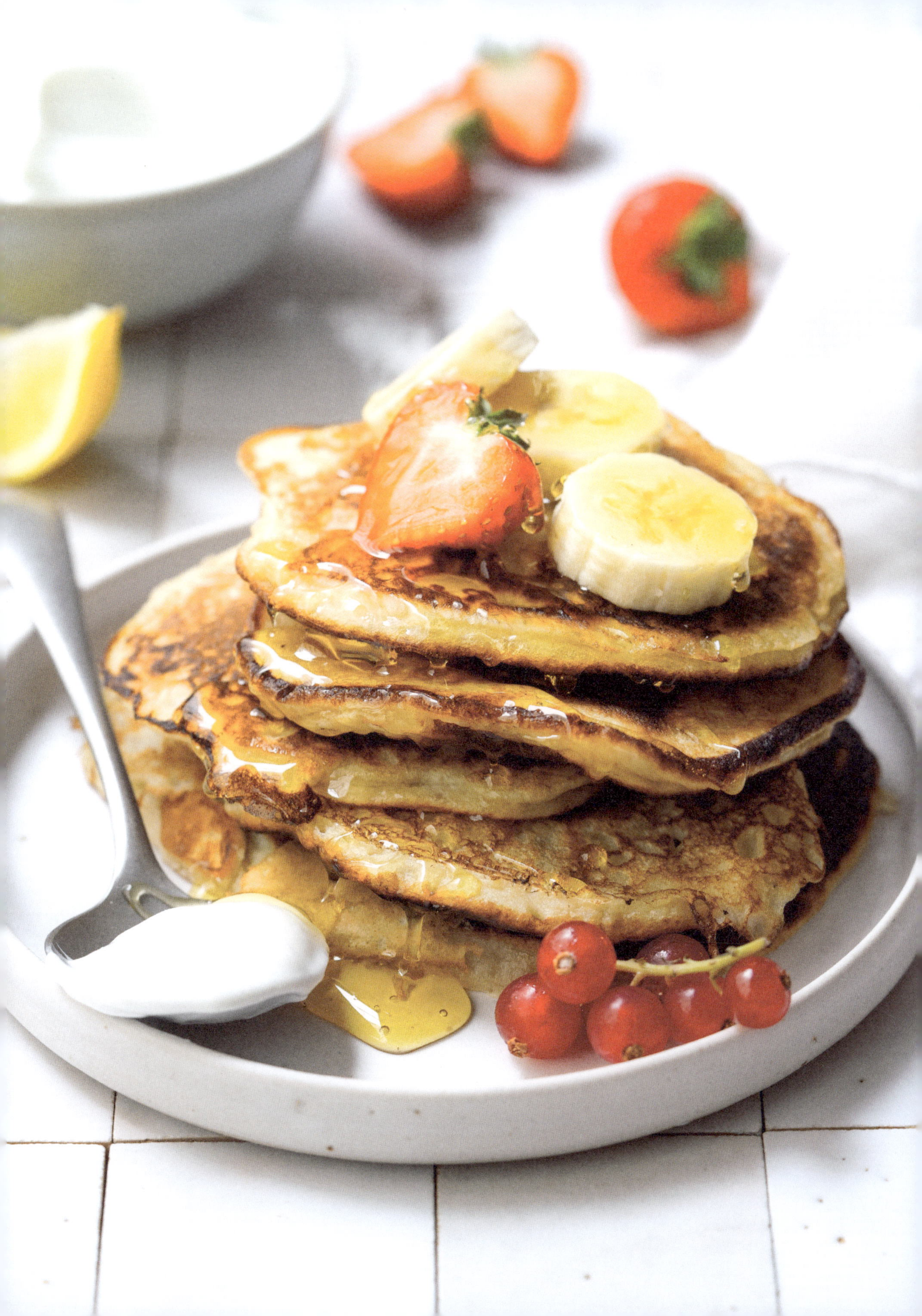

Pulled Pork Burgers

As a supplement

To boost production

SERVES **2** • PREPARATION TIME: **20 MINUTES** • COOKING TIME: **3¼ HOURS**
RESTING TIME: **1 HOUR**

4 burger buns
1 Little Gem lettuce
150 g (5 oz) mixed raw vegetables (carrots, red and white cabbage), finely grated
coriander leaves, to garnish

FOR THE PICKLED RED ONION

4 tablespoons white vinegar
120 ml (4 fl oz) water
30 g (1¼ oz) caster sugar
½ red onion, thinly sliced

FOR THE PULLED PORK

3 tablespoons sunflower oil
600 g (1 lb 5 oz) diced pork shoulder
120 g (4 oz) honey
240 g (8½ oz) barbecue sauce
100 ml (3½ fl oz) soy sauce
400 ml (14 fl oz) beef stock
1 tablespoon smoked paprika
1½ teaspoons ground cumin
1½ teaspoons dried oregano
4 garlic cloves, finely chopped

FOR THE SPICY MAYO

4 tablespoons mayonnaise
1 tablespoon Sriracha sauce
1 tablespoon lime juice

1. First, make the pickled red onion. In a small pan, bring the vinegar, water and sugar to the boil. Once the sugar has dissolved, add the sliced red onion. Remove from the heat and set aside to rest, then place in a jar in the refrigerator for at least 1 hour.
2. Next, prepare the pulled pork. Heat the oil in a casserole dish. When hot, sauté the pork for 5 minutes, then add the remaining ingredients and bring to the boil. Reduce the heat, cover and cook for 3 hours, stirring occasionally.
3. Once cooked, shred the meat using 2 forks and set it aside in its juices.
4. Combine the spicy mayo ingredients in a bowl.
5. Cut the buns in half and place them, cut-sides up, under a hot grill to toast for a few minutes.
6. Spread the toasted buns with spicy mayo, add some lettuce leaves, grated vegetables, pickled red onion, pulled pork and coriander leaves and sandwich together.

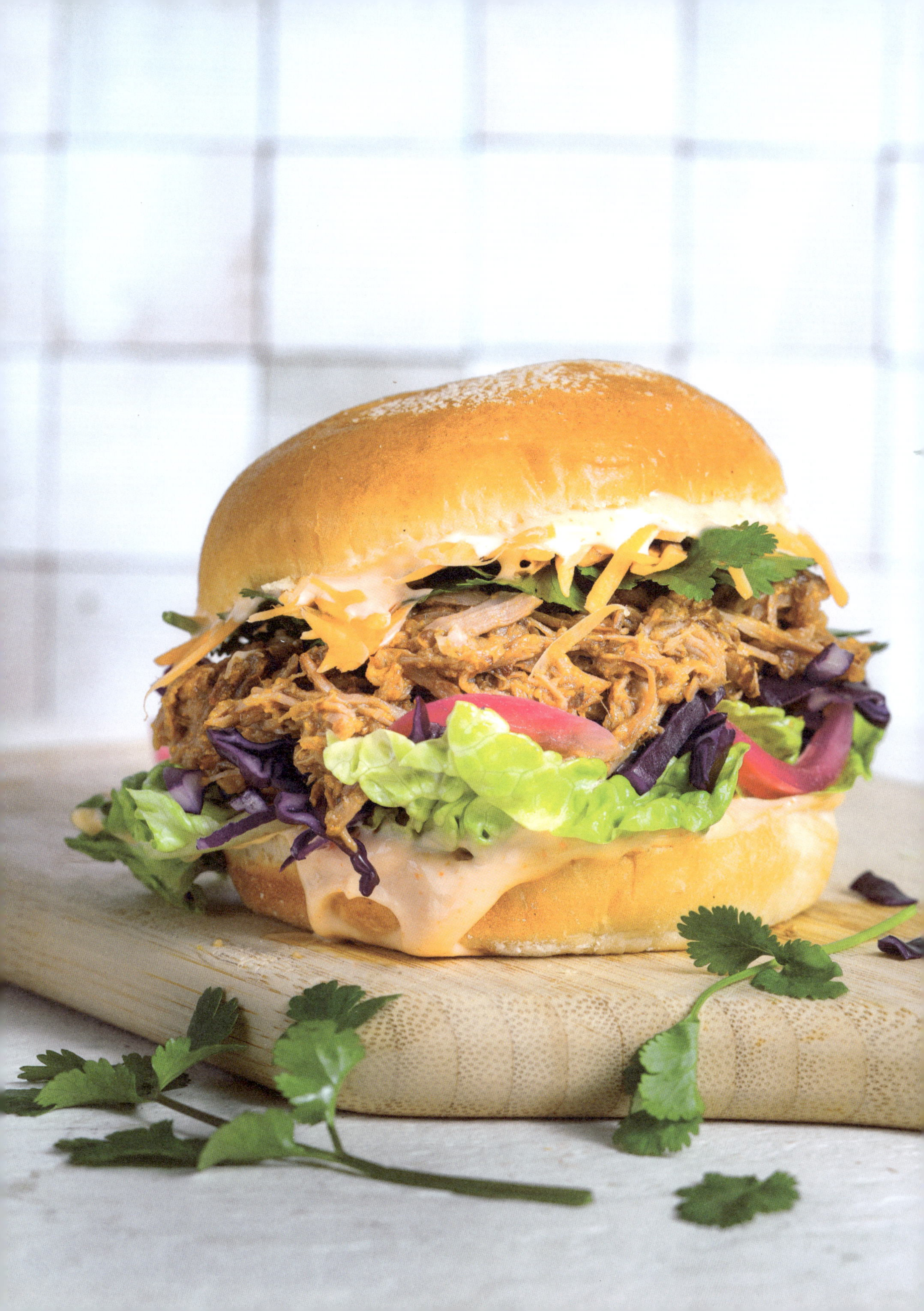

To boost production

Sweet Potatoes Stuffed with Lamb

SERVES **2** • PREPARATION TIME: **10 MINUTES** • COOKING TIME: **1 HOUR**

FOR THE ROASTED CHICKPEAS

250 g (8 oz) drained canned chickpeas
2 tablespoons olive oil
2 teaspoons curry powder
pinch of salt

FOR THE SWEET POTATOES

2 medium sweet potatoes, washed
2 tablespoons sunflower oil

FOR THE HUMMUS

150 g (5 oz) drained canned chickpeas
juice of ½ lemon
1 tablespoon tahini
100 ml (3½ fl oz) hot water
salt and pepper

FOR THE LAMB

250 g (8 oz) shredded lamb (from 7-Hour French-style 'Spoon' Lamb, see page 34)
a few spoonfuls of stock
50 ml (2 fl oz) olive oil
2 garlic cloves, thinly sliced
2 handfuls of baby spinach
salt and pepper

TO GARNISH

40 g (1½ oz) pine nuts
6 chives, finely chopped

1. Preheat the oven to 200°C (400°F), Gas Mark 6.
2. Combine the chickpeas with the oil, curry powder and salt. Place on a baking sheet lined with baking paper and bake in the oven for 30 minutes.
3. Prick the sweet potatoes with the tip of a small, sharp knife and bake in the oven for 45 minutes–1 hour, depending on their size, until soft all the way through.
4. Meanwhile, make the hummus. In a blender, blend the chickpeas with the lemon juice, tahini, hot water and a pinch each of salt and pepper.
5. For the lamb, reheat the meat in a saucepan with a few spoonfuls of stock for about 15 minutes over a medium heat, with the lid on.
6. Heat the oil in a separate small saucepan, then add the garlic and gently fry for a few minutes. Add the baby spinach and stir until wilted.
7. Cut open the sweet potatoes lengthways, separating the two halves. Crush them lightly in the centre with the back of a spoon, then top with the hummus, lamb, spinach and garlic, a sprinkle of roasted chickpeas and some pine nuts and chives.

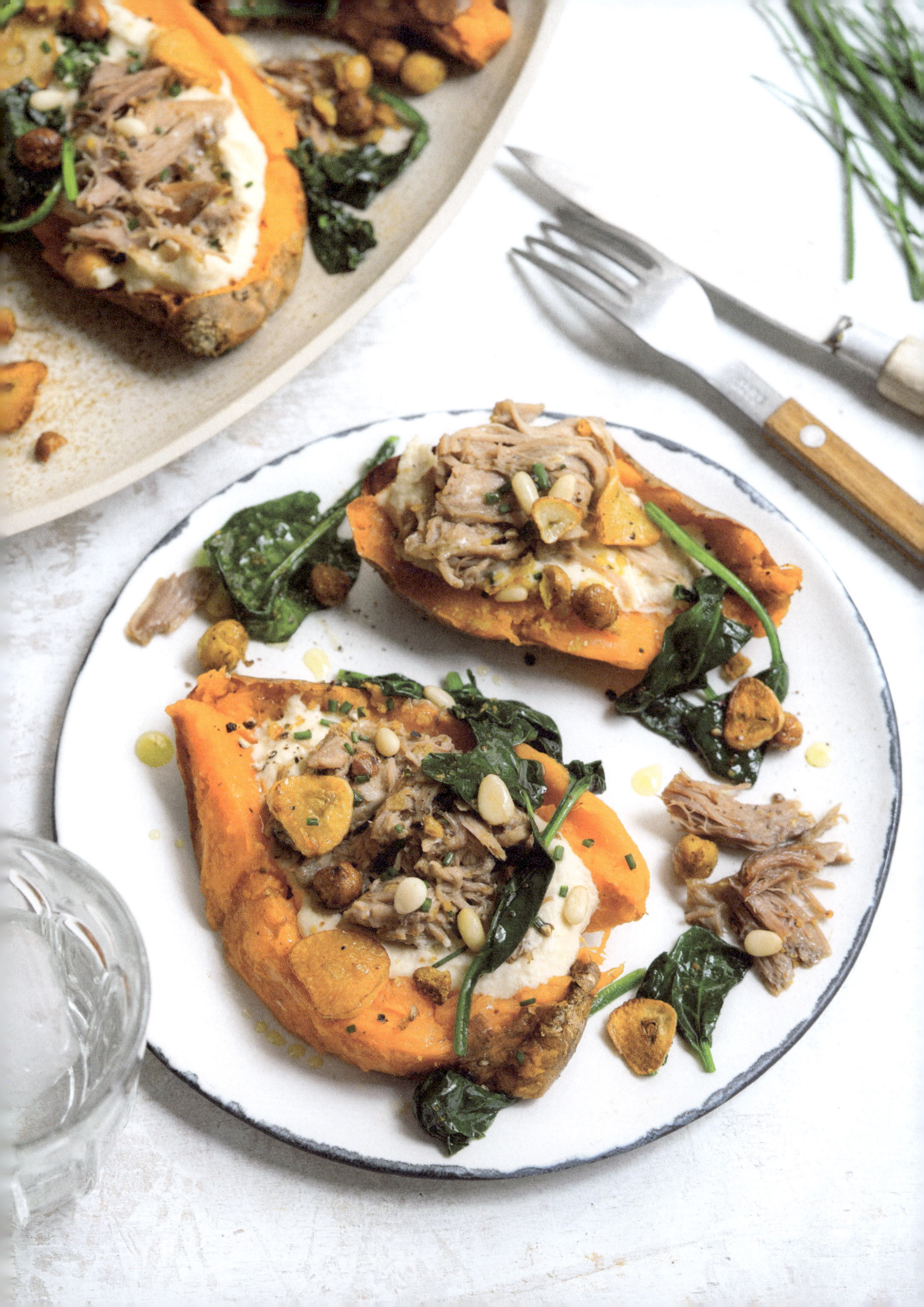

As a supplement

To boost production

Aguadito, Peruvian-style Chicken and Rice Soup

SERVES **2** • PREPARATION TIME: **20 MINUTES** • COOKING TIME: **30 MINUTES**

1 tablespoon olive oil
½ onion, finely chopped
1 garlic clove, finely chopped
1 carrot, peeled and sliced
1 red chilli, finely chopped
1 pre-cooked corn on the cob, cut into 4 slices
1 chicken breast fillet (or 150 g/5 oz shredded chicken from making the Chicken Stock; see page 16)
800 ml (28 fl oz) Chicken Stock (see page 16)
30 g (1¼ oz) rice
80 g (3 oz) frozen broad beans (or peas)
leaves from 4 coriander sprigs
½ avocado, thinly sliced
1 lime, cut into wedges

1. Heat the oil in a large saucepan. When hot, sauté the onion, garlic, carrot and chilli in the oil for 3 minutes. Add the slices of corn and shredded chicken to the pan and pour in the stock. Cover and simmer for 15 minutes.
2. Add the rice and cook for a further 5 minutes.
3. Add the broad beans (or peas) and cook for a final 7 minutes.
4. Add the coriander leaves and sliced avocado before serving with a few lime wedges.

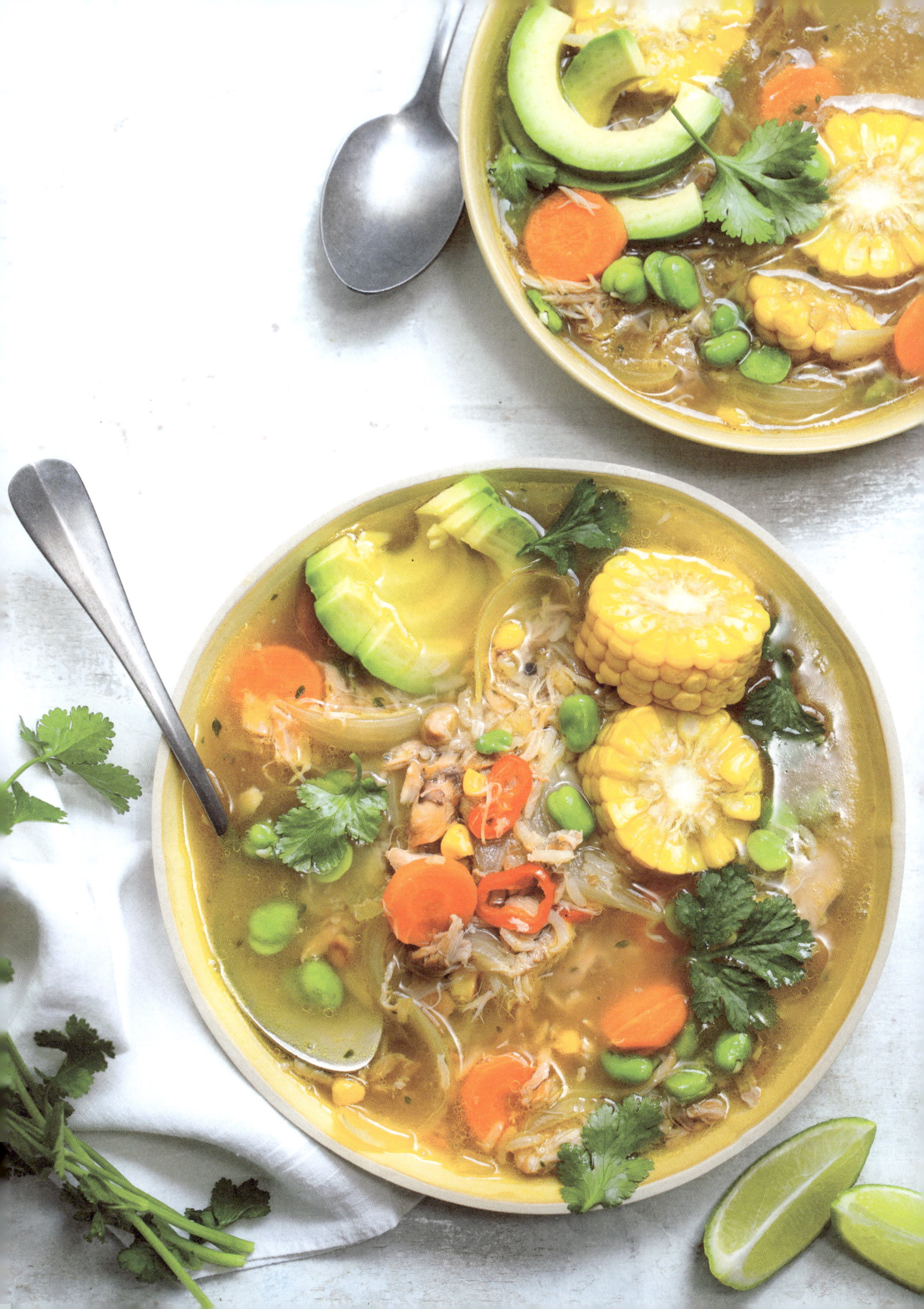

As a supplement

To boost production

Traditional 'Pot-au-Feu' Stew

SERVES **2** • PREPARATION TIME: **35 MINUTES** • COOKING TIME: **1 HOUR**
RESTING TIME: **1½ HOURS**

1 recipe quantity of French-style 'Pot-au-Feu' Broth (see page 17), vegetables and meat reserved

2 marrow bones

coarse salt

300 g (10 oz) potatoes, peeled

¼ green cabbage, rinsed and outer leaves removed, cut into wedges

2 turnips, peeled and cut into wedges

wholegrain mustard, to serve

1. Soak the marrow bones in a large bowl of cold water salted with coarse salt. Place in the refrigerator for about 1½ hours, while you carry on with the rest of the recipe.
2. Place the potatoes in a saucepan of salted cold water and bring to the boil. Cook for 20–25 minutes.
3. Meanwhile, bring 1 litre (1¾ pints) of the 'Pot-au-Feu' Broth to the boil. Cook the cabbage in the broth for 15 minutes, then add the turnip wedges and cook for another 15 minutes.
4. Add the reserved 'Pot-au-Feu' meat and continue to cook over a medium heat for about 20 minutes, covered with the lid.
5. Drain the marrow bones and place in a saucepan of fresh water salted with coarse salt. Bring to the boil and cook for 10 minutes, then remove from the heat and leave to rest for 10 minutes.
6. Serve the 'Pot-au-Feu' meat with the marrow bones, vegetables and a small amount of wholegrain mustard.

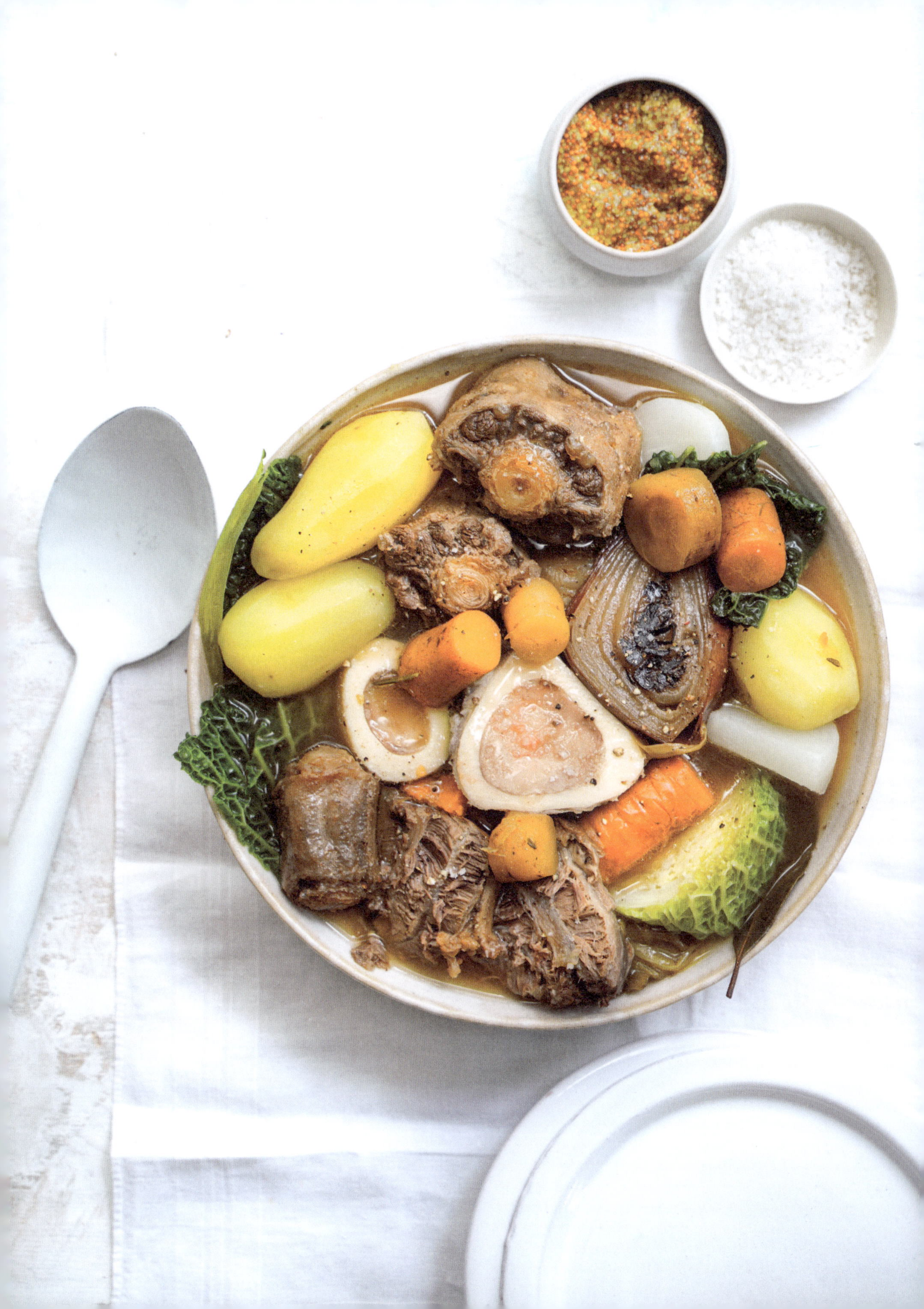

As a supplement

To boost production

Vibrant Watercress Soup

SERVES **2** • PREPARATION TIME: **10 MINUTES** • COOKING TIME: **25 MINUTES**

FOR THE SOUP

1 bunch of watercress
20 g (¾ oz) butter
1 shallot, finely chopped
150 g (5 oz) potatoes, peeled and diced
500 ml (17 fl oz) Chicken Stock (see page 16)
100 ml (3½ fl oz) double cream
salt and pepper

FOR THE TOPPINGS

2 slices of smoked trout, chopped
handful of sprouted seeds
1 teaspoon pink peppercorns, crushed
drizzle of soya cream (optional)

1. Remove the damaged parts of the watercress stems, then wash the leaves and stems separately. Finely chop the stems.
2. Melt the butter in a saucepan, then sweat the shallot, watercress stems and potatoes for 2 minutes over a medium heat. Season with salt and pepper, then pour in the chicken stock. Cover and simmer for 20 minutes.
3. Bring another large pan of salted water to the boil. Add the watercress leaves and blanch for 3 minutes, then drain and refresh in a bowl of cold water. Drain again.
4. Check whether the potatoes are cooked, then transfer the contents of the saucepan to a blender. Blend until smooth.
5. Empty the blender jug and add the watercress leaves and cream. Blend until you have a bright green purée, then add this to the soup mixture, stirring well.
6. Serve the soup with the chopped smoked trout, some sprouted seeds, a pinch of crushed pink peppercorns and a dash of soya cream, if desired.

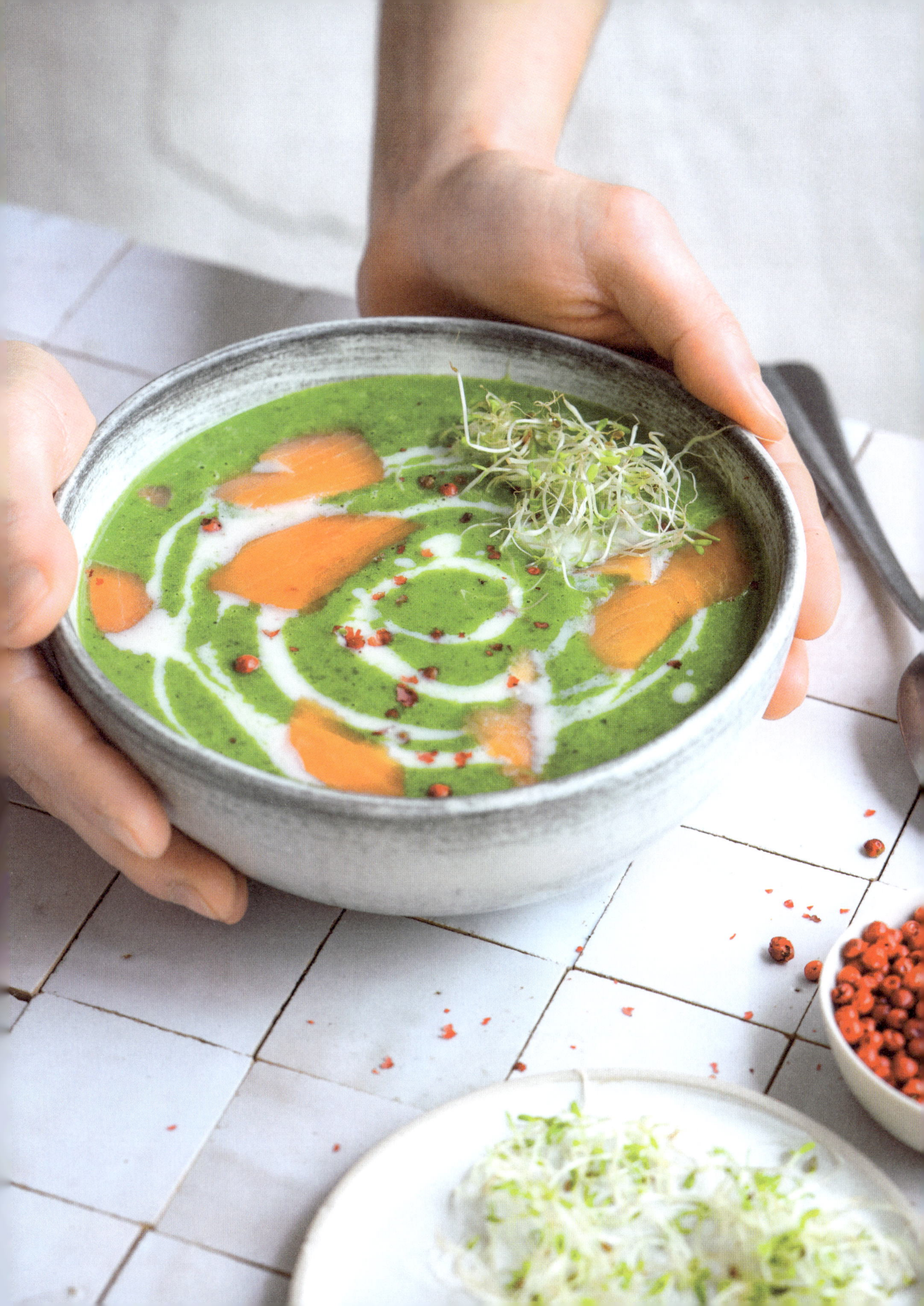

As a supplement

To boost production

Forest Fruits Gravlax Smorgasbord

SERVES **2** • PREPARATION TIME: **20 MINUTES** • COOKING TIME: **5 MINUTES**
RESTING TIME: **OVERNIGHT**

FOR THE GRAVLAX

1 piece of boneless, skin-on salmon (about 350 g/ 11 ½ oz)
40 g (1 ½ oz) white sugar
60 g (2 ¼ oz) coarse salt
1 tablespoon pink peppercorns, crushed
100 g (3 ½ oz) frozen blueberries
100 g (3 ½ oz) frozen blackcurrants (or redcurrants)
50 g (2 oz) frozen raspberries
250 ml (8 fl oz) water

FOR THE PICKLED RED ONION

½ red onion, thinly sliced
20 g (¾ oz) caster sugar
40 ml (1 ½ fl oz) white vinegar
80 ml (3 fl oz) water

TO SERVE

8 slices of toasted Nordic seed bread
200 g (7 oz) fromage frais
1 mini cucumber (or ½ cucumber), finely chopped
12 radishes, finely sliced
a few dill sprigs, chopped
juice of 1 lemon

1. To make the gravlax, combine the sugar, salt and crushed peppercorns in a bowl.
2. In a small blender, blend all the frozen fruit with the measured water. Add to the sugar, salt and peppercorn mixture and mix well.
3. Place half the mixture in an airtight container. Place the piece of salmon on top and push gently down into the mixture. Pour the rest of the mixture on top. Place in the refrigerator overnight (or for up to 24 hours).
4. To make the pickled red onion, place the sliced onion in an airtight container or a glass jar. Mix the sugar, vinegar and measured water in a small saucepan and bring to the boil. As soon as the sugar has dissolved, pour the hot liquid over the onion. Seal and store overnight in the refrigerator.
5. The next day, remove the fish from its marinade and wipe dry with a kitchen towel before cutting into slices.
6. Spread the toasted bread with the fromage frais and garnish with the cucumber, radishes, pickled onions, fish slices and dill. Add a squeeze of lemon juice before enjoying.

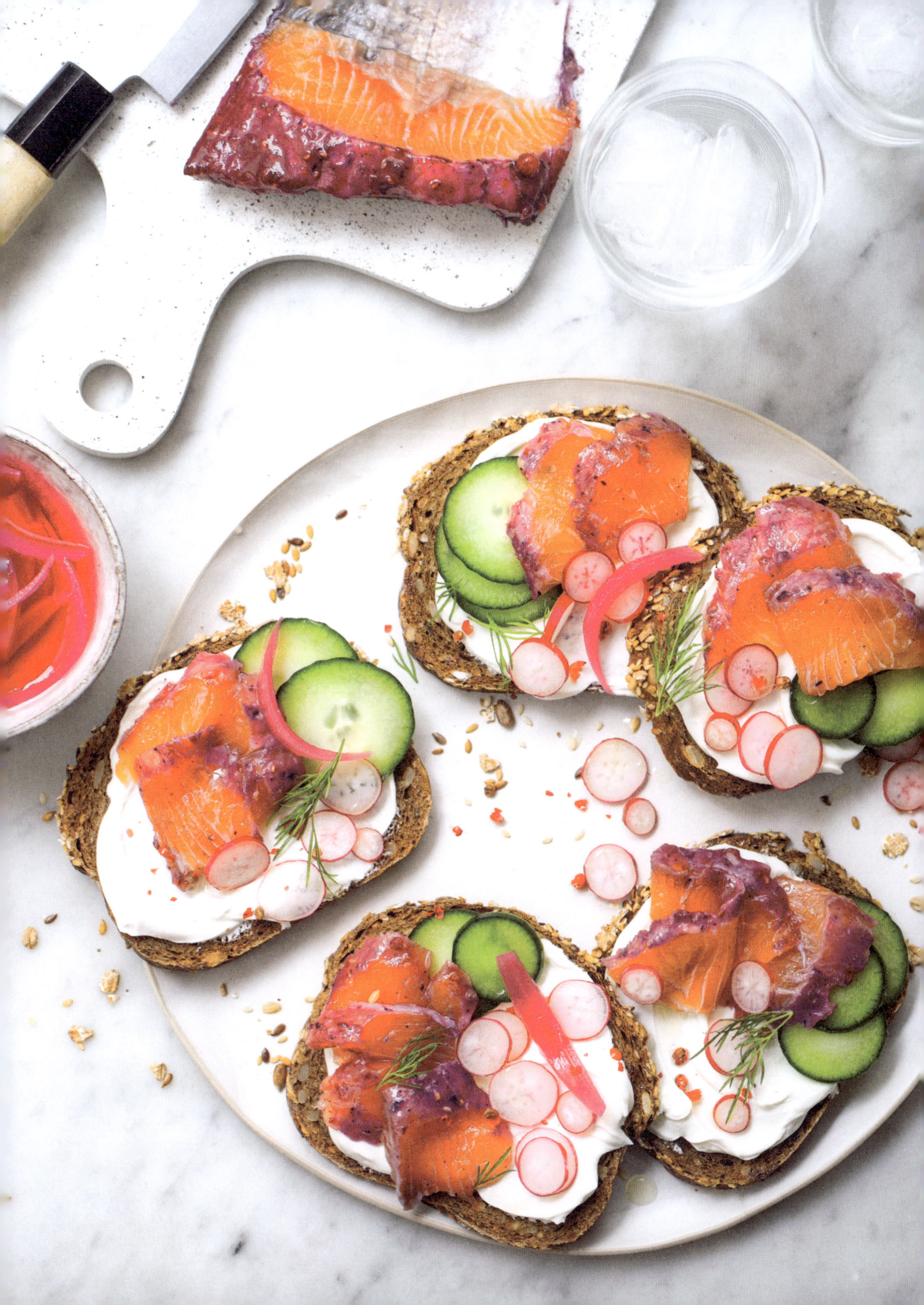

Lentil and Squash Dhal

SERVES **2** • PREPARATION TIME: **15 MINUTES** • COOKING TIME: **30 MINUTES**

splash of oil
½ onion, finely chopped
2 garlic cloves, finely chopped
10 g (½ oz) fresh root ginger, peeled and finely chopped
1 teaspoon Colombo spice powder (mild Caribbean or French-style curry powder)
1 teaspoon ground turmeric
120 g (4 oz) red lentils
150 g (5 oz) canned crushed tomatoes
½ squash, deseeded and thickly sliced (with the skin on)
400 ml (14 fl oz) Vegetable Stock (see page 23)
150 ml (5 fl oz) coconut cream
5 coriander sprigs, chopped
pinch of black sesame seeds
salt and pepper

1. Heat the oil in a saucepan. When hot, sauté the onion, garlic, ginger and spices for 2 minutes, then add the lentils, crushed tomatoes, squash slices and Vegetable Stock. Cover and simmer for 15 minutes.
2. Add the coconut cream and cook for a further 12 minutes.
3. Adjust the seasoning and serve with a sprinkle of chopped coriander and black sesame seeds.

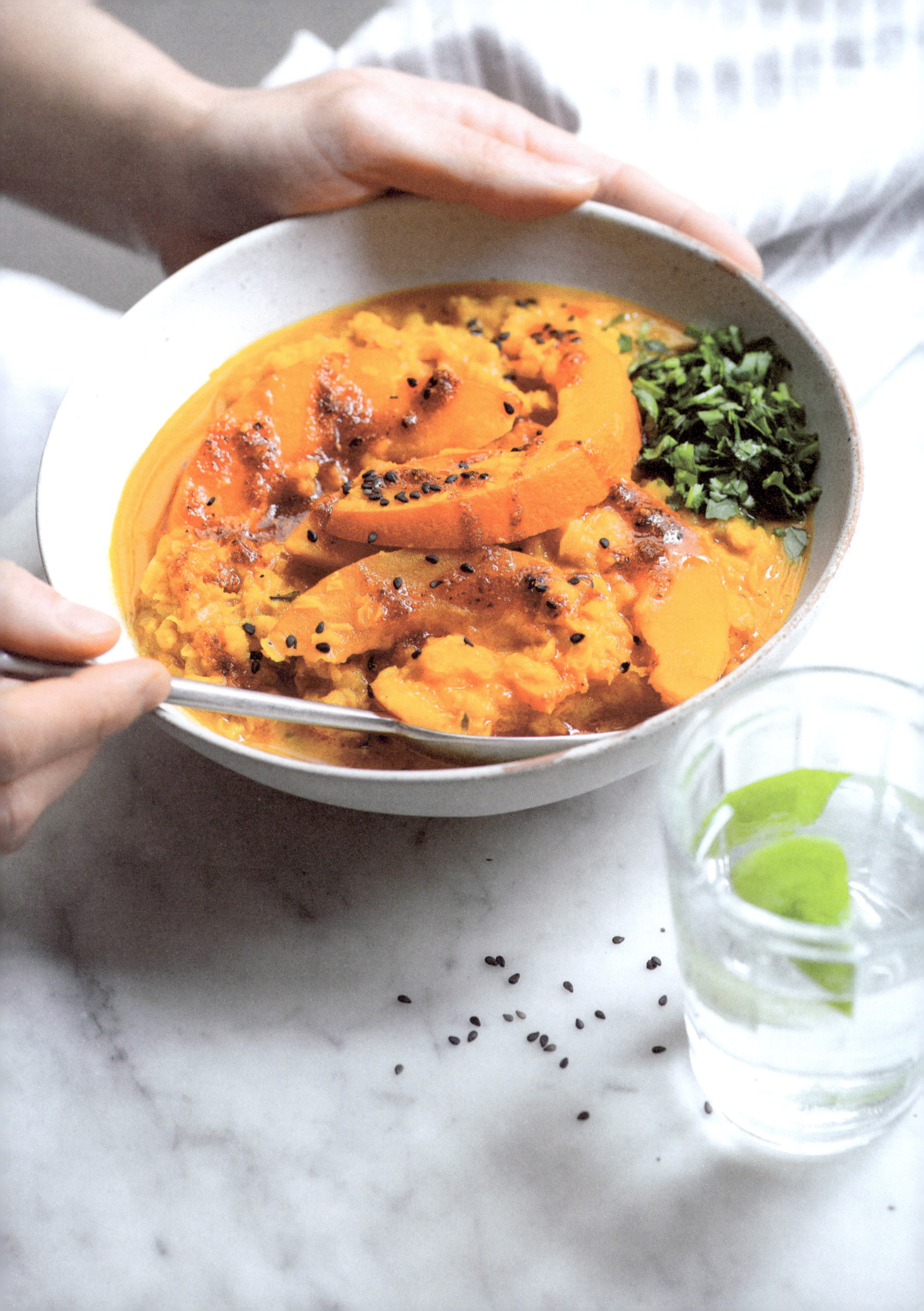

COLLAGEN THERAPY • AUTUMN

Joint recovery and strengthening

Autumn is the perfect season to strengthen the joints and stimulate collagen production in the connective tissues. Priority is given to amino acids, proteins and minerals.

AIM

To strengthen the joints, bones and muscles before winter.

KEY NUTRIENTS

To stimulate collagen production naturally, some essential cofactors are required.

- **Vitamin C** (citrus fruit, red berries, peppers, parsley and broccoli)
- **Zinc and copper** (oysters, seeds, dark chocolate, cashew nuts, sunflower seeds, lean red meat)
- **Omega-3 fatty acids** (oily fish, avocado, flaxseed)
- **Antioxidants** (green tea, berries, raw cacao, carrots, turmeric)

Things to know

- **For anti-inflammatory action:** turmeric, ginger, green tea, oily fish
- **To strengthen the bones:** enriched plant-based milks, Brazil nuts, sunflower seeds, kale, almonds, bananas, broccoli

KEY FOODS

The following foods contain bioactive collagen and essential amino acids for connective tissue reconstruction.

- **Fish,** including the skin and bones (salmon, sardines, mackerel)
- **Chicken** (skin and cartilage)
- **Bone broth** (beef, chicken, fish)
- **Egg white** (rich in proline, a precursor to collagen)
- **Pork rind** (baked, jellied, in homemade pâté)
- **Natural gelatine and collagen powder**

	DAY 1	DAY 2
BREAKFAST	Pink Beetroot Latte • see page 27 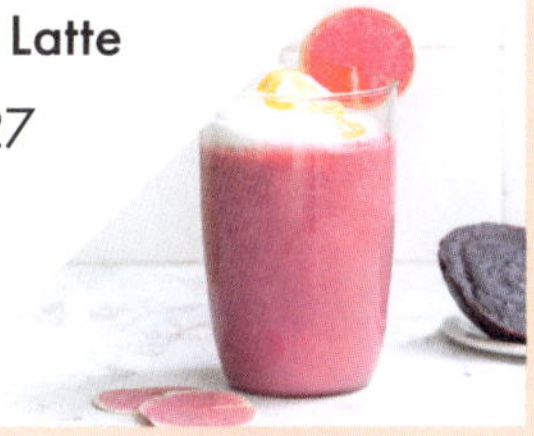	Chocolate and Banana Oatmeal Porridge • see page 124 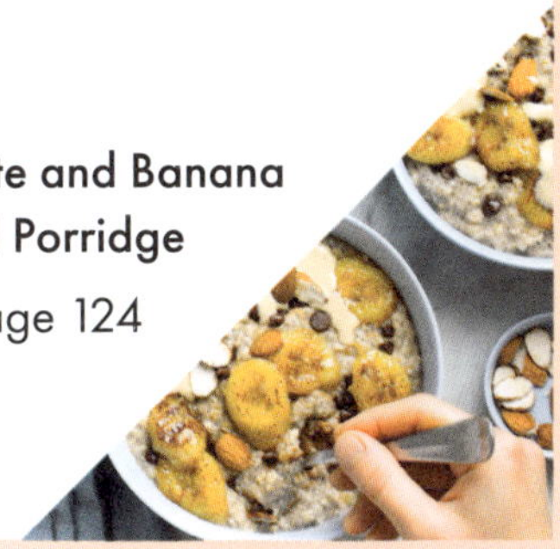
LUNCH	Pulled Pork Burgers • see page 94 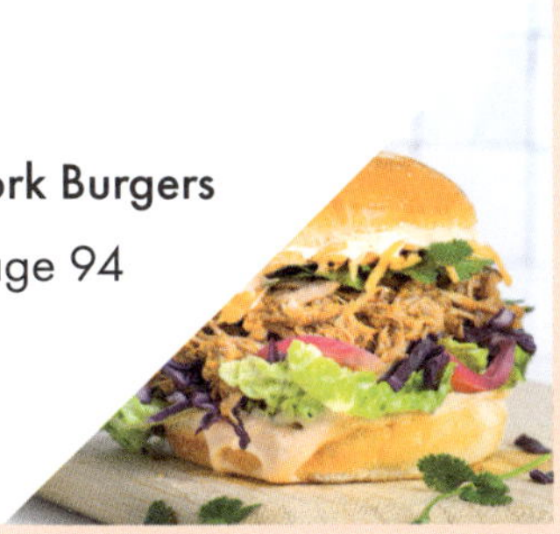	Traditional 'Pot-au-Feu' Stew • see page 100 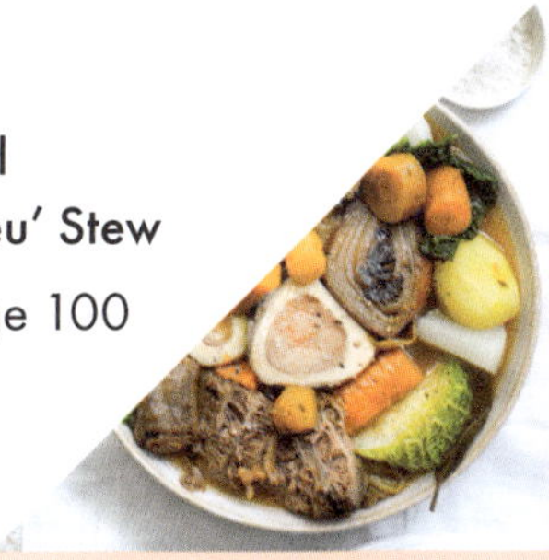
SNACK	Coconut and Mango Flan • see page 150 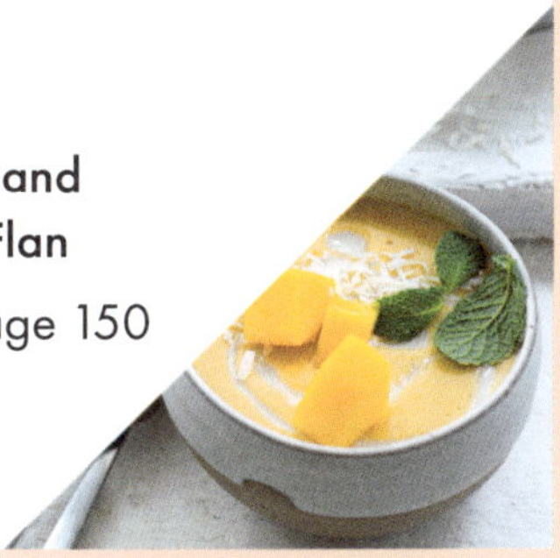	Golden Latte • see page 28 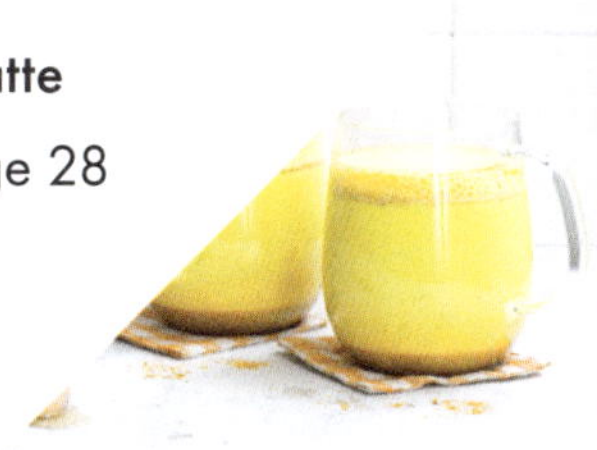
DINNER	**Roast pork and root vegetables** (sweet potatoes, turnips, carrots): place a pork tenderloin in a casserole dish with the peeled and chopped vegetables, drizzle over a little olive oil, cover and cook for about 30 minutes at 170°C (350°F), Gas Mark 4	Pearl Barley Minestrone with Squash • see page 148 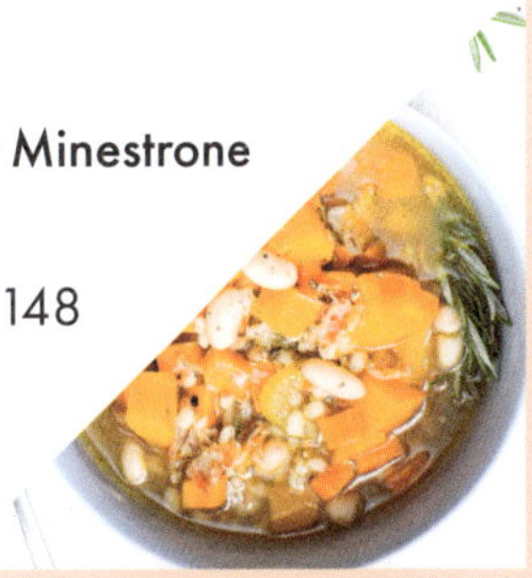

As a supplement

To boost production

Fish Ramen

SERVES **2** • PREPARATION TIME: **25 MINUTES** • COOKING TIME: **20 MINUTES**
RESTING TIME: AT LEAST **2 HOURS**

FOR THE PICKLED EGGS

2 eggs
50 ml (2 fl oz) soy sauce
40 ml (1½ fl oz) mirin
1 tablespoon sugar
60 ml (2½ fl oz) Dashi (see page 22)

FOR THE RAW MARINATED MACKEREL

2 mackerel fillets
50 g (2 oz) sugar
70 g (2¾ oz) coarse salt

FOR THE BROTH

2 salted anchovies
1 garlic clove, finely chopped
1 tablespoon miso
800 ml (28 fl oz) Fish Stock (see page 20) or Dashi (see page 22)
4 shiitake or button mushrooms

TO SERVE

150 g (5 oz) buckwheat (or wholewheat) noodles
handful of baby spinach
8 slices of Daikon radish (white) or Red Meat radish (pink)

1. Cook the eggs for 6 minutes in a saucepan of boiling water until soft-boiled. Place the eggs immediately in a bowl of cold water to stop the cooking process. Carefully peel the eggs and place them in an airtight plastic bag filled with all the pickling ingredients. Place in the refrigerator for at least 2 hours (or up to 24 hours).
2. Rinse and dry the mackerel fillets. Mix the sugar and salt in a bowl. Slash 3 cuts in the skin of each fillet and place in the curing mixture for about 1 hour. After this time, remove the mackerel fillets from the bowl and wipe off the salt and sugar cure with kitchen paper, or rinse with cold water.
3. Meanwhile, to make the broth, heat the anchovies, garlic and miso in a saucepan for a few minutes. Crush to a paste, then cover with the Fish Stock or Dashi. Add the mushrooms and simmer for 10 minutes.
4. Cook the noodles according to the packet instructions.
5. Divide the noodles, cured mackerel fillets, spinach and radishes between 2 large bowls. Cover with boiling hot broth, then garnish with the halved eggs.

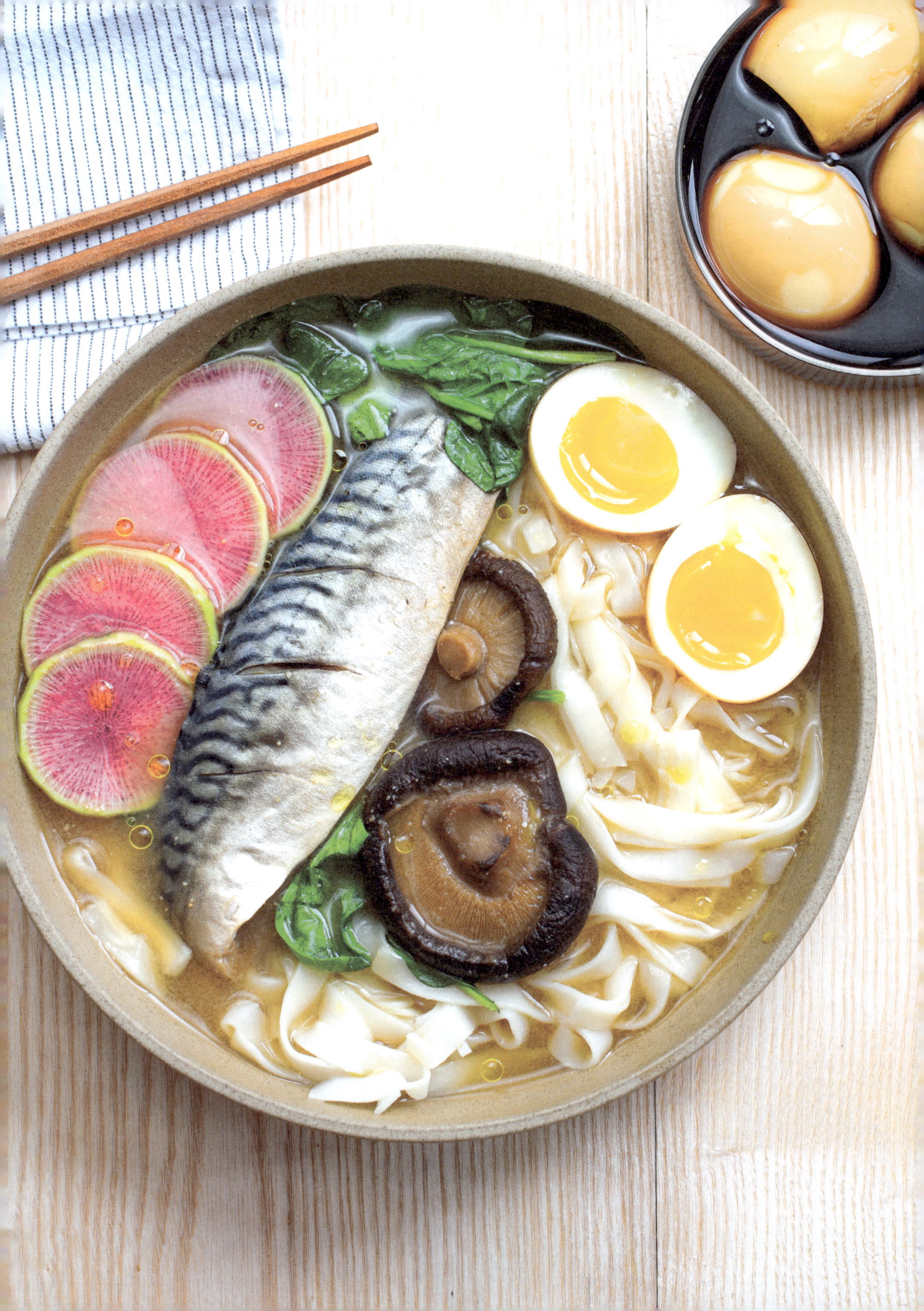

Tuna, Fennel and Citrus Salad

SERVES **2** • PREPARATION TIME: **15 MINUTES** • COOKING TIME: **30 MINUTES**

100 g (3½ oz) bulgur wheat
1 orange
2 clementines
70 g (2¾ oz) rocket leaves
1 tablespoon olive oil
2 tuna steaks

FOR THE ROAST VEGETABLES

2 celery sticks, cut into 3–4 cm (1½ inch) pieces
1 fennel bulb, halved and sliced into thin wedges
1 tablespoon olive oil
salt and pepper

FOR THE ORANGE VINAIGRETTE

juice of 1 orange
juice of 1 lemon
3 tablespoons rapeseed oil
salt and pepper

1. Cook the bulgur wheat according to the packet instructions.
2. Preheat the oven to 200°C (400°F), Gas Mark 6.
3. Place the celery and fennel in an ovenproof dish. Drizzle with the olive oil and add a pinch of salt and pepper. Mix well. Bake in the oven for 25–30 minutes.
4. Meanwhile, peel the orange and clementines. Slice between the pith to remove the orange segments and cut the clementines widthways into slices (reserving all the juices released).
5. To prepare the vinaigrette, mix the citrus juices (including the reserved juice) with the rapeseed oil and a pinch each of salt and pepper.
6. Combine the roasted vegetables with the bulgur wheat, citrus pieces and rocket in a salad bowl. Drizzle with the vinaigrette and toss.
7. Heat the olive oil in a frying pan. When hot, fry the tuna steaks for 30 seconds on each side until medium-rare, then cut into thick slices. Serve with the citrus salad.

Tip

You can also sprinkle crushed pistachios over the salad.

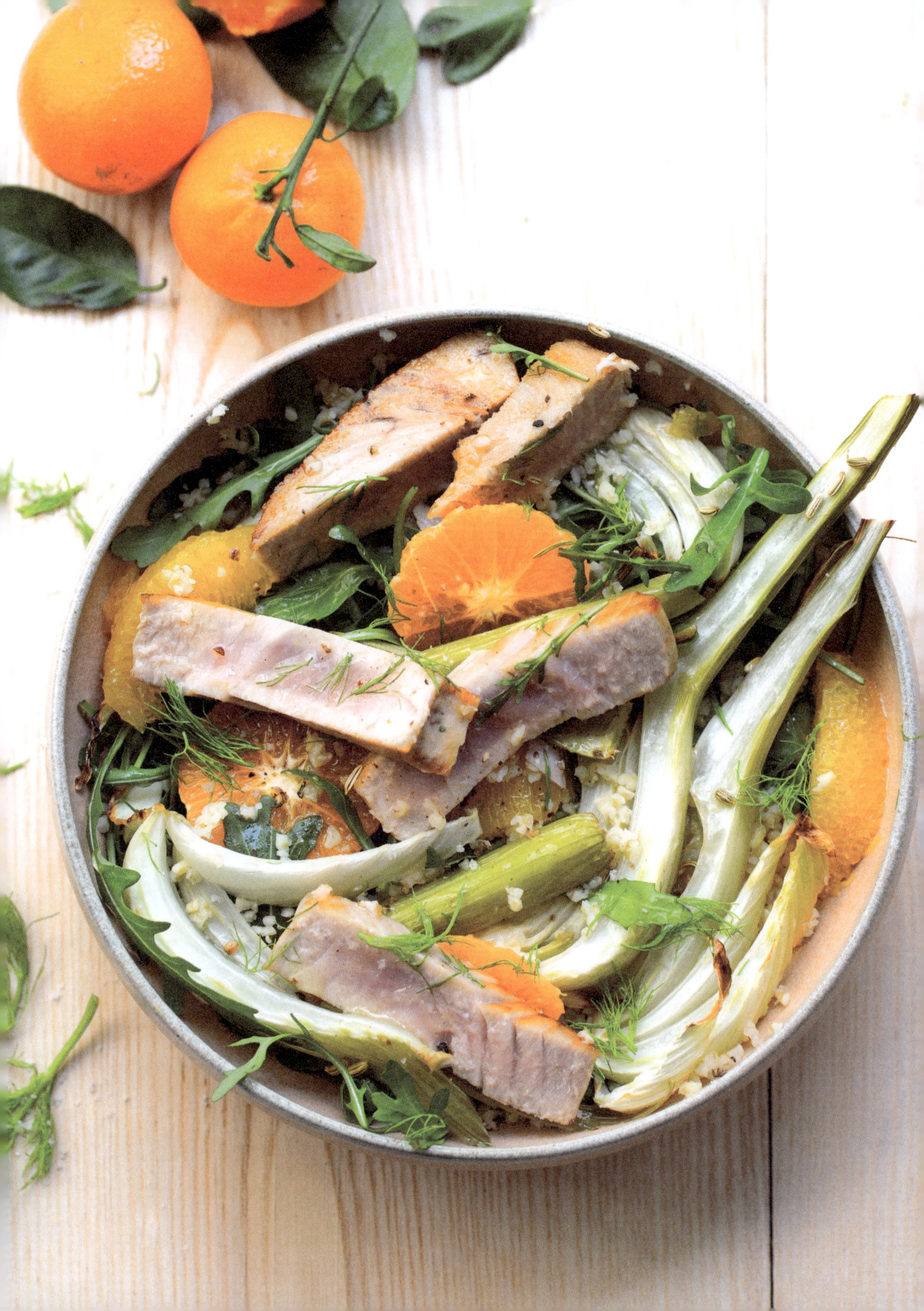

To boost production

Kimchi Stew

SERVES **2** • PREPARATION TIME: **10 MINUTES** • COOKING TIME: **20 MINUTES**

200 g (7 oz) good-quality kimchi
1 tablespoon sunflower oil
½ onion, finely chopped
1 garlic clove, finely chopped
3 fresh shiitake or button mushrooms, sliced
500 ml (17 fl oz) Vegetable Stock (see page 23) or Dashi (see page 22)
pinch of chilli powder (or 1 teaspoon chilli paste)
250 g (8 oz) firm tofu, cut into bite-sized cubes
120 g (4 oz) rice noodles
2 tablespoons soy sauce
1 spring onion, finely sliced
salt and pepper

1. Strain the kimchi and reserve the juices.
2. Heat the oil in a casserole dish. When hot, sauté the onion and garlic for 3 minutes, then add the kimchi and mushrooms. Cook for 1 minute.
3. Cover with the stock and add the chilli powder, kimchi juice and tofu. Season with salt and pepper, cover and simmer for 15 minutes.
4. Meanwhile, cook the noodles separately according to the packet instructions.
5. Once the stew has cooked, add the soy sauce and spring onion and divide between 2 bowls filled with the noodles.

Tip

For a non-vegetarian version, add 100 g (3½ oz) minced pork, sautéed at the same time as the onion and garlic.

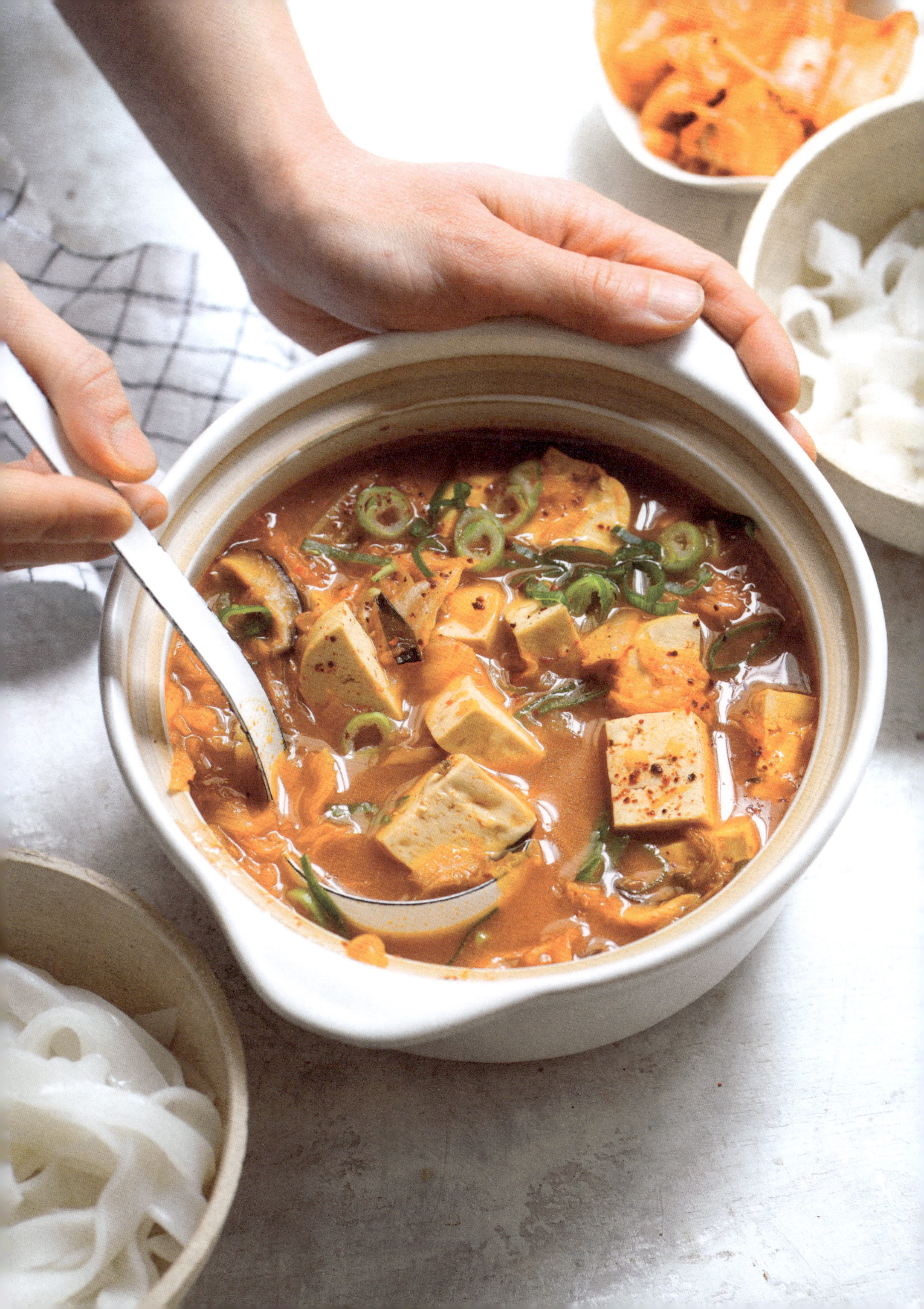

Citrus Quinoa Salad with Marinated Prawns

To **boost** production

SERVES **2** • PREPARATION TIME: **20 MINUTES** • COOKING TIME: **16 MINUTES**

100 g (3½ oz) tricolour quinoa
1 grapefruit
1 blood orange (or 1 regular orange)
150 g (5 oz) cooked shelled prawns
2 tablespoons olive oil
½ teaspoon za'atar
1 avocado, pitted, peeled and cut into slices
2 tablespoons goji berries
35 g (1¼ oz) pecans or Brazil nuts
2 handfuls of lamb's lettuce
1 burrata
salt

FOR THE VINAIGRETTE

juice of ½ lemon
5 tarragon sprigs, finely chopped
50 ml (2 fl oz) olive oil
salt and pepper

1. Cook the quinoa in a large saucepan of salted boiling water according to the packet instructions. Leave to cool.
2. Peel the grapefruit and blood orange and cut into thin slices.
3. To make the vinaigrette, mix the lemon juice with the tarragon, oil and some salt and pepper.
4. Mix the prawns with 1 tablespoon of the olive oil and the za'atar.
5. Heat the remaining tablespoon of oil in a non-stick pan. Fry the avocado slices for about 30 seconds on each side, then remove from the pan. Add the prawns to the pan and fry for 5 minutes.
6. Mix all the ingredients together, dress with the vinaigrette and serve immediately with the burrata on the side.

Tip

If you don't have za'atar, mix ½ teaspoon ground cumin with ½ teaspoon dried Provençal herbs and 1 teaspoon sesame seeds.

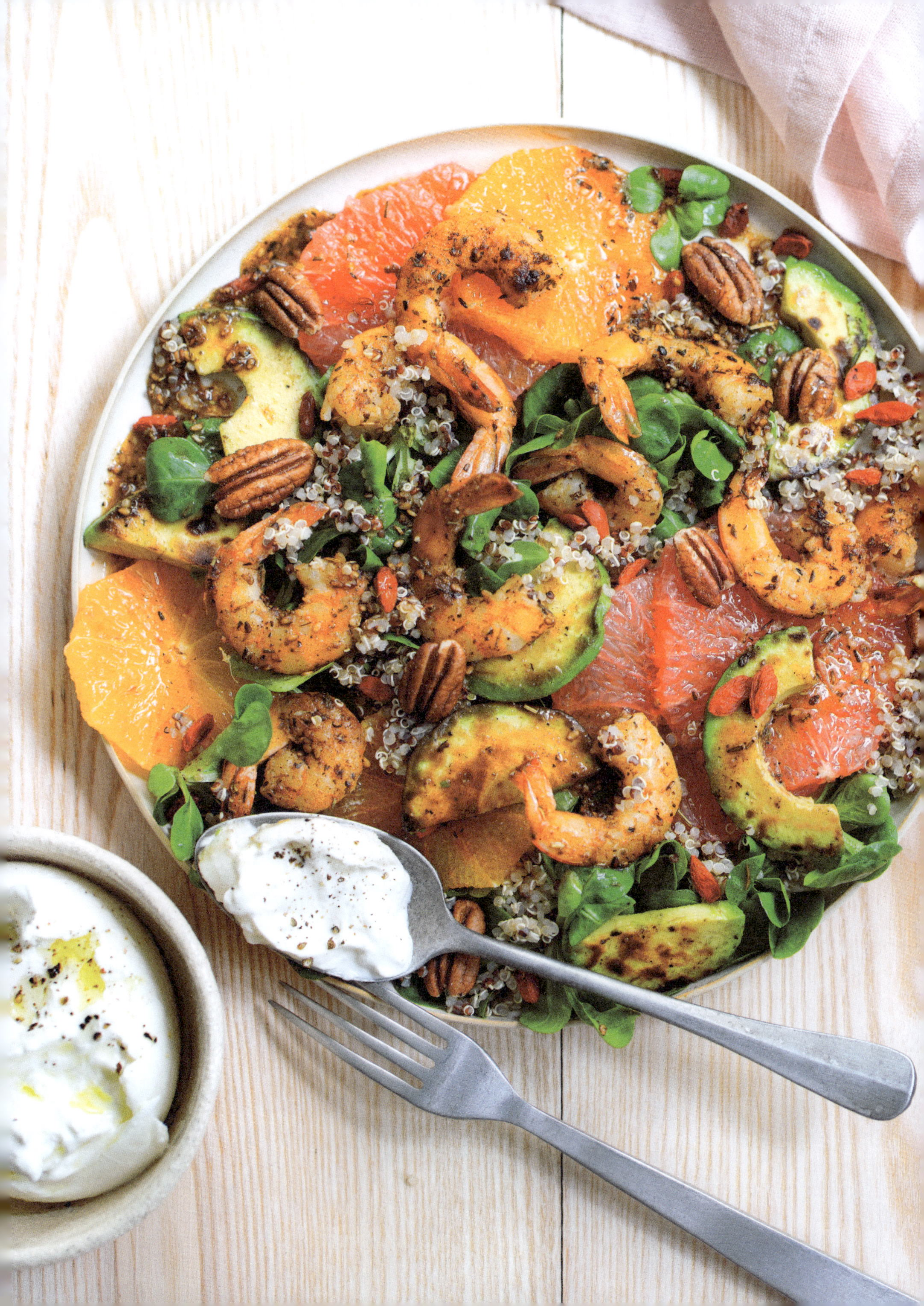

To boost production

Chickpea Curry

SERVES **2** • PREPARATION TIME: **15 MINUTES** • COOKING TIME: **25 MINUTES**

1 tablespoon sunflower oil
½ brown onion, finely chopped
1 garlic clove, finely chopped
2 teaspoons curry powder (or 1 teaspoon yellow curry paste)
½ teaspoon ground turmeric
250 g (8 oz) drained canned chickpeas
200 g (7 oz) canned crushed tomatoes
300 ml (½ pint) Vegetable Stock (see page 23)
300 ml (½ pint) coconut milk
½ red onion, thinly sliced
juice of ½ lime
7 coriander sprigs, finely chopped
150 g (5 oz) red rice
40 g (1 ½ oz) baby spinach
30 g (1 ¼ oz) cashew nuts
salt and pepper

1. Heat the oil in a saucepan over a medium heat. When hot, sauté the onion and garlic for 3 minutes, then add the spices and cook for 1 minute.
2. Add the chickpeas, crushed tomatoes and stock and simmer for 10 minutes.
3. Add the coconut milk and cook for a further 10 minutes.
4. In a bowl, mix the sliced onion with the lime juice and three-quarters of the chopped coriander.
5. Meanwhile, cook the rice according to the packet instructions.
6. Once the curry is cooked, add the baby spinach and stir until wilted. Season to taste.
7. Serve the curry with the drained rice, garnished with the remaining chopped coriander, marinated red onion and the cashew nuts.

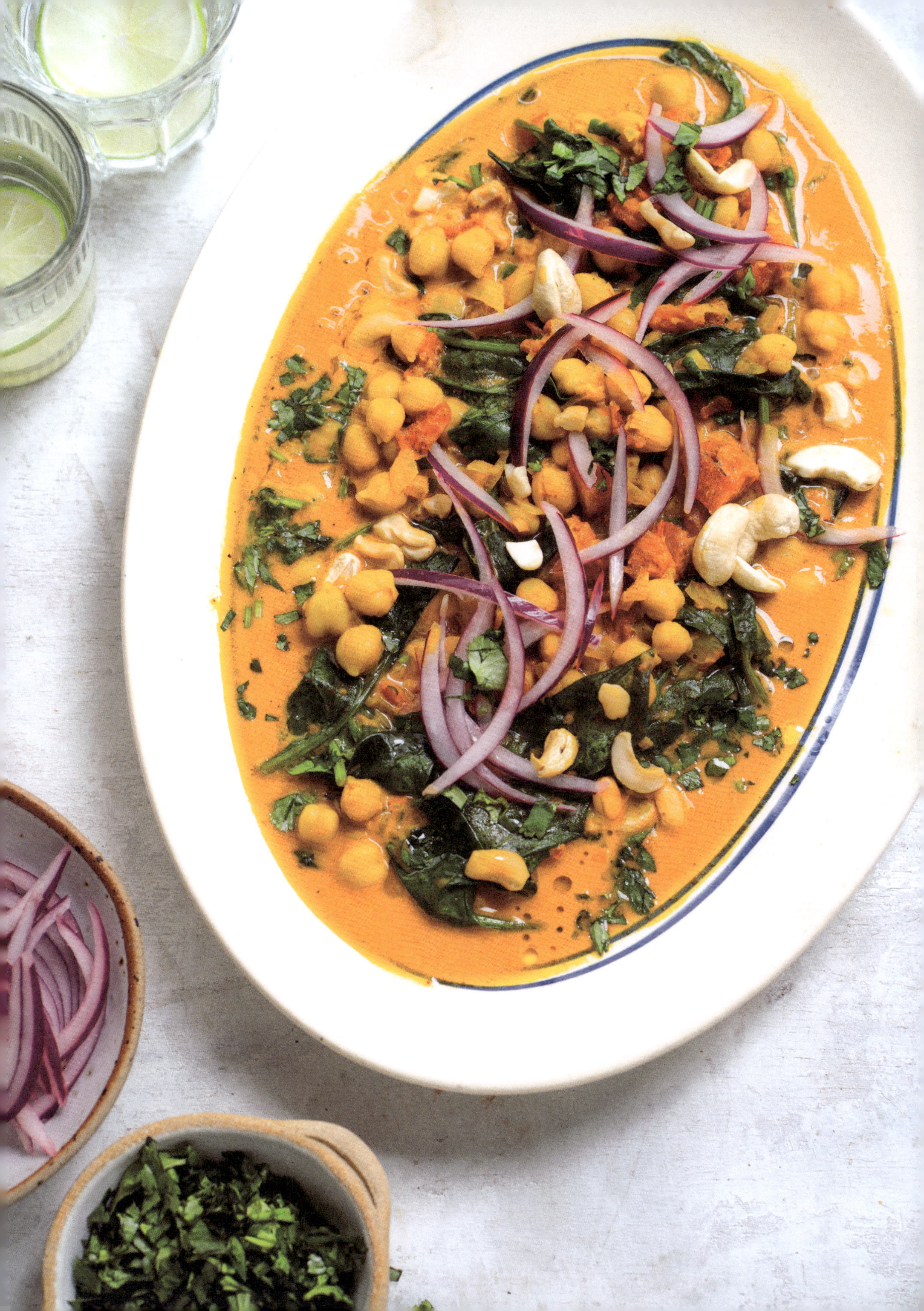

Chocolate Fondant Squares

SERVES **8** • PREPARATION TIME: **20 MINUTES** • COOKING TIME: **20 MINUTES**
RESTING TIME: **2 HOURS**

FOR THE BROWNIE

100 g (3½ oz) milk chocolate
2 eggs
40 g (1½ oz) brown sugar
10 g (½ oz) unsweetened cocoa powder (or raw cacao)
25 g (1 oz) plain flour
35 g (1½ oz) ground almonds
1 teaspoon baking powder
100 g (3½ oz) courgette (about ½ courgette), grated
pinch of sea salt flakes

FOR THE FUDGE LAYER

80 g (3 oz) dark chocolate
55 g (2¼ oz) peanut butter (or almond butter)
180 ml (6 fl oz) coconut milk

1. Preheat the oven to 180°C (350°F), Gas Mark 4.
2. For the brownie, melt the chocolate in a microwave or bain-marie.
3. In a bowl, beat together the eggs and sugar, then add the melted chocolate, cocoa, flour, ground almonds and baking powder. Beat thoroughly until you have a smooth paste, then incorporate the grated courgette with a spatula.
4. Tip the mixture into a square or rectangular cake tin lined with baking paper (leave an overhang to help with unmoulding). Bake in the oven for 15–20 minutes (or until an inserted skewer comes out clean).
5. Remove from the oven and let cool.
6. To make the fudge layer, melt the dark chocolate and peanut butter in the coconut milk. Pour the mixture over the brownie and place in the refrigerator for at least 2 hours.
7. Remove from the tin by carefully lifting out the baking paper, then cut into squares. Sprinkle with sea salt flakes before serving.

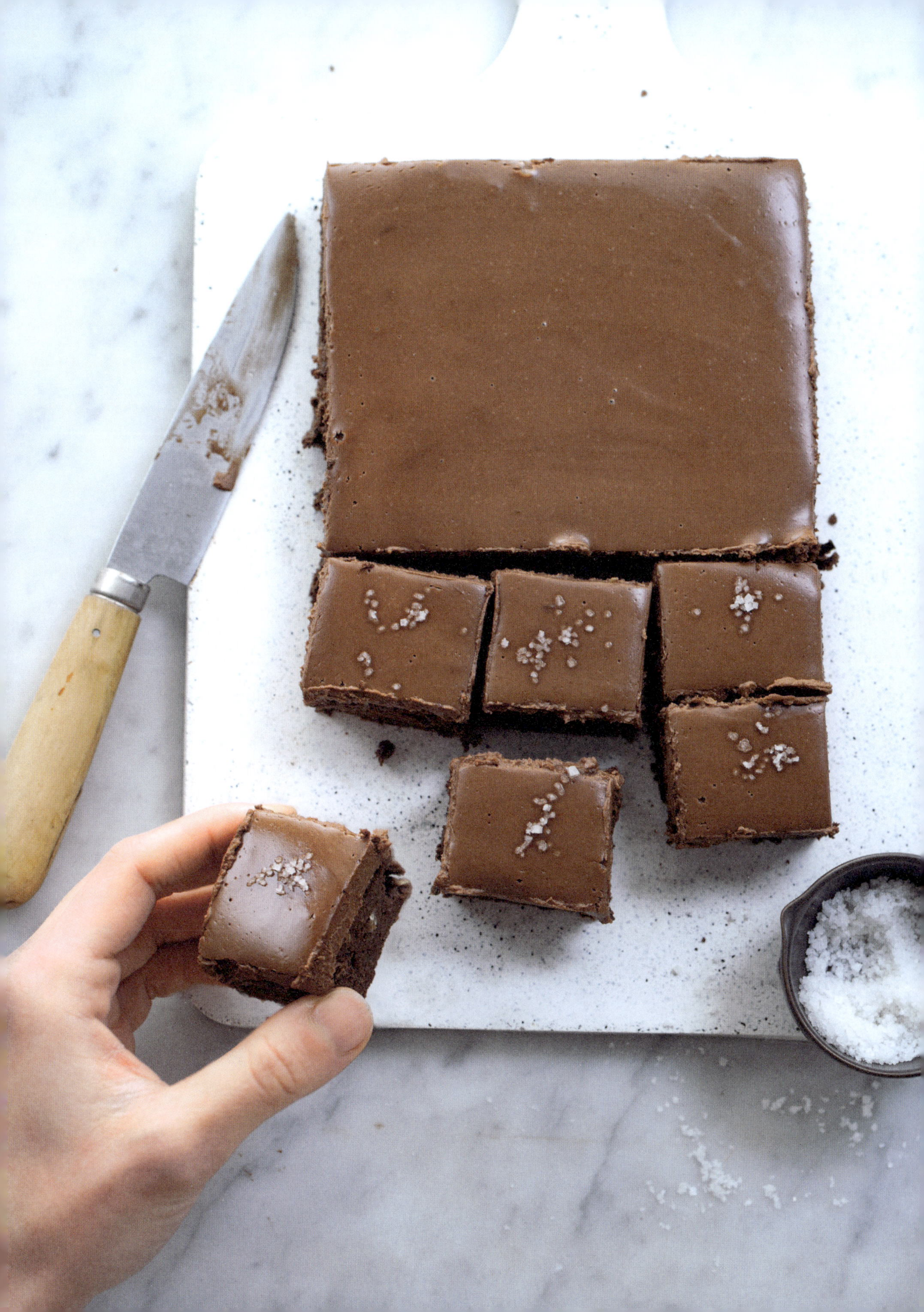

Seasonal Tips

Eat collagen-rich stews to benefit from easily absorbed and warming nutrients.

Combine collagen sources with citrus fruit and vitamin C-rich vegetables to maximize their assimilation.

Combine probiotics and fibre to strengthen gut flora and improve the absorption of nutrients.

Combine collagen + vitamin C + probiotics + Omega-3 in every meal for an immunity boost, easier digestion and radiant skin all winter.

Drink a ginger and turmeric infusion to combat inflammation and boost collagen production.

Winter Recipes

To **boost** production

Chocolate and Banana Oatmeal Porridge

SERVES **2** • PREPARATION TIME: **5 MINUTES** • COOKING TIME: **15 MINUTES**

3 bananas
100 g (3½ oz) porridge oats
3 tablespoons chia seeds
550 ml (17½ fl oz) oat milk
pinch of vanilla powder or ground cinnamon (according to taste)
pinch of sea salt flakes
1 tablespoon coconut oil
1 tablespoon unrefined brown cane sugar
2 tablespoons almond butter
40 g (1½ oz) dark chocolate chips (75% cocoa solids)
handful of almonds

1. Peel one of the bananas and mash with a fork.
2. In a saucepan, combine the mashed banana with the porridge oats, chia seeds, oat milk, flavouring of choice and the salt. Bring to the boil and cook for 10 minutes over a medium heat, stirring from time to time.
3. Slice the remaining bananas.
4. Heat the coconut oil and sugar in a frying pan over a high heat, add the sliced bananas and caramelize for 2 minutes.
5. Pour the porridge into 2 bowls and top with the almond butter, caramelized bananas, chocolate chips and a few almonds.

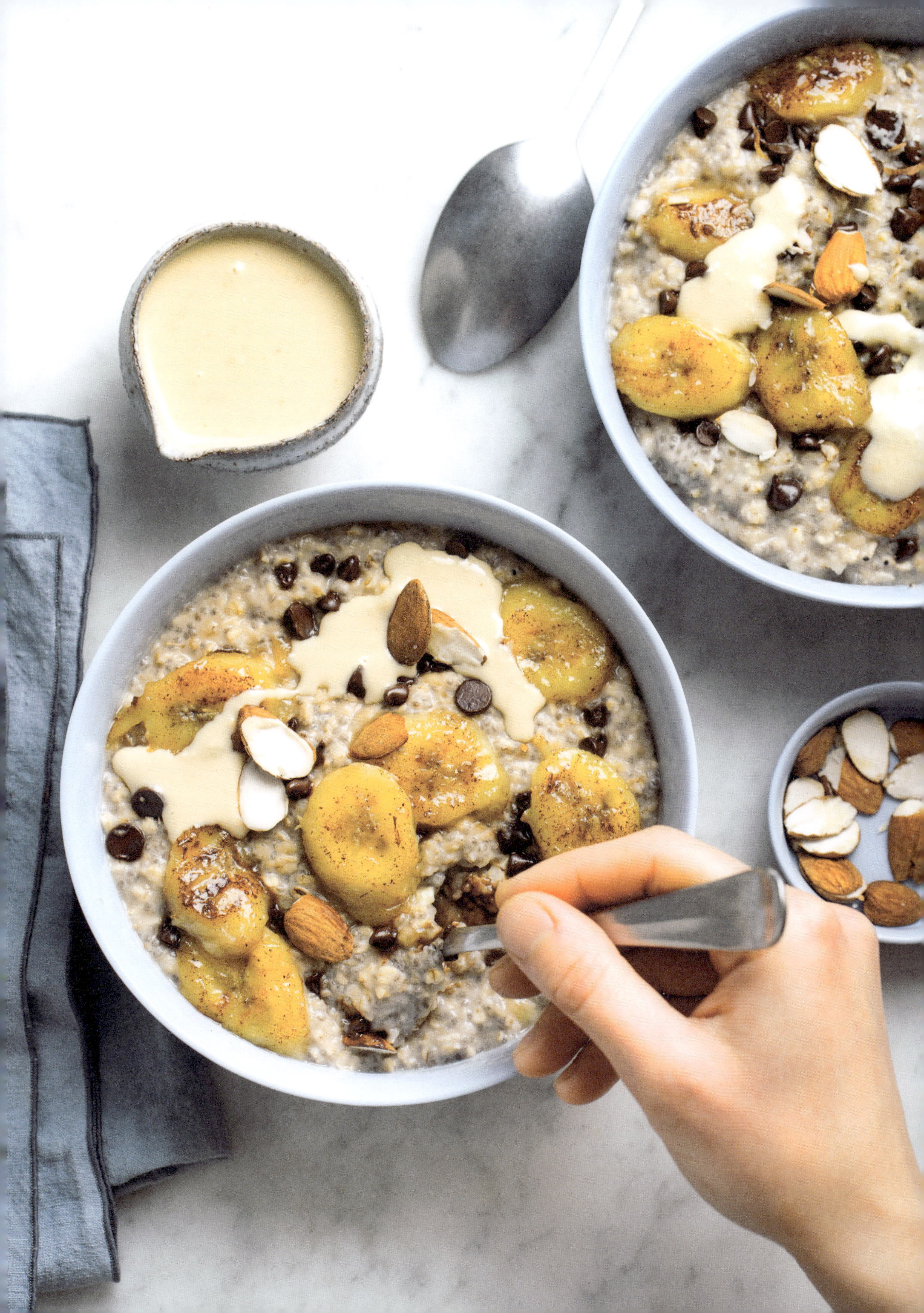

As a supplement

To boost production

Chorba

SERVES **2** • PREPARATION TIME: **10 MINUTES** • COOKING TIME: **1½–1¾ HOURS**

1 tablespoon olive oil
2 garlic cloves, peeled and halved
1 onion, finely chopped
250 g (8 oz) saddle of lamb (sliced through the bone) (or shredded leftovers from the 7-Hour Lamb recipe on page 34), cut into large bite-sized pieces
1 celery stick, thinly sliced
1 carrot, peeled and thinly sliced
2 tablespoons concentrated tomato paste
1 tablespoon ras el hanout
700 ml (24 fl oz) lamb, chicken or beef stock
1 leek (white part only), washed and thinly sliced
100 g (3½ oz) drained canned chickpeas
8 chives, finely chopped
salt and pepper

1. Heat the oil in a casserole dish. When hot, sauté the garlic and onion for 2 minutes, then add the lamb pieces along with the central bone. Cook for a further 3 minutes.
2. Add the celery, carrot, tomato paste and spices. Season and pour in the stock. Cover and cook over a low heat for 1–1¼ hours.
3. Add the leek and chickpeas and continue to cook with the lid on for a further 20 minutes.
4. Check the tenderness of the meat – it should come apart easily. Serve garnished with the chopped chives.

Tip

You can make your own tagine spice mix by combining 1 teaspoon garam masala, 1 teaspoon ground cumin, ½ teaspoon ground coriander and ½ teaspoon ground nutmeg.

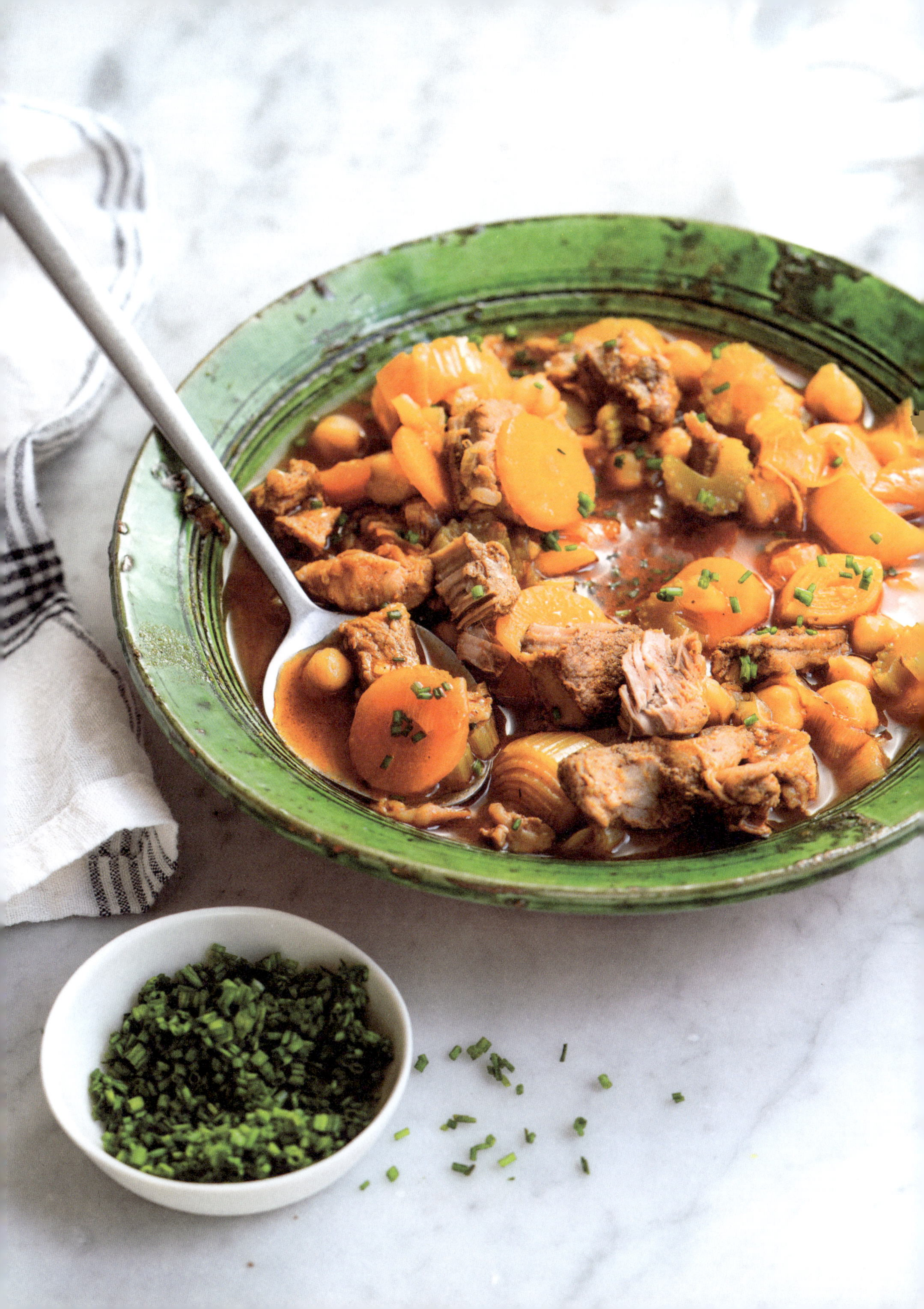

Chicken, Carrot and Sweet Potato Parmentier

As a supplement

To boost production

SERVES **2** • PREPARATION TIME: **25 MINUTES**
COOKING TIME: **1 HOUR 10 MINUTES**

FOR THE SWEET POTATO AND CARROT PURÉE

150 g (5 oz) carrots, peeled and chopped
350 g (11 ½ oz) sweet potatoes, peeled and chopped
salt and pepper

FOR THE MEAT

250 g (8 oz) leftover shredded chicken meat (from the Stock recipe on page 16) plus a few cooked vegetables from the stock
5 chervil sprigs, chopped, plus extra to garnish
salt and pepper

FOR THE SAVOURY PARMESAN CRUMBLE

60 g (2¼ oz) butter
75 g (3 oz) plain flour
60 g (2¼ oz) Parmesan cheese (or Grana Padano), grated
½ teaspoon ground turmeric

1. Preheat the oven to 200°C (400°F), Gas Mark 6.
2. Start with the sweet potato and carrot purée. Place the carrots and sweet potatoes in a large saucepan of salted water, bring to the boil, cover and cook for 25 minutes.
3. In a saucepan, reheat the shredded chicken and vegetables with a few spoonfuls of stock for about 15 minutes over a low heat. Add the chopped chervil and some salt and pepper, then tip the mixture into a gratin dish.
4. Drain the carrots and sweet potatoes and mash with a potato masher or fork. Season with salt and pepper and spread the mash over the meat layer in the gratin dish.
5. Mix all the crumble ingredients to a crumbly dough, then sprinkle over the top of the mash. Bake in the oven for 30 minutes.
6. Serve garnished with a few extra chervil sprigs.

Tip

If you don't have any pre-prepared stock or cooked meat, place 3 chicken thighs in the saucepan with 2 carrots and 1 celery stick, cut into chunks, and cook at a simmer for 35–40 minutes until the thighs are tender. The collagen content will, however, be lower than in a stock that has been cooked over several hours.

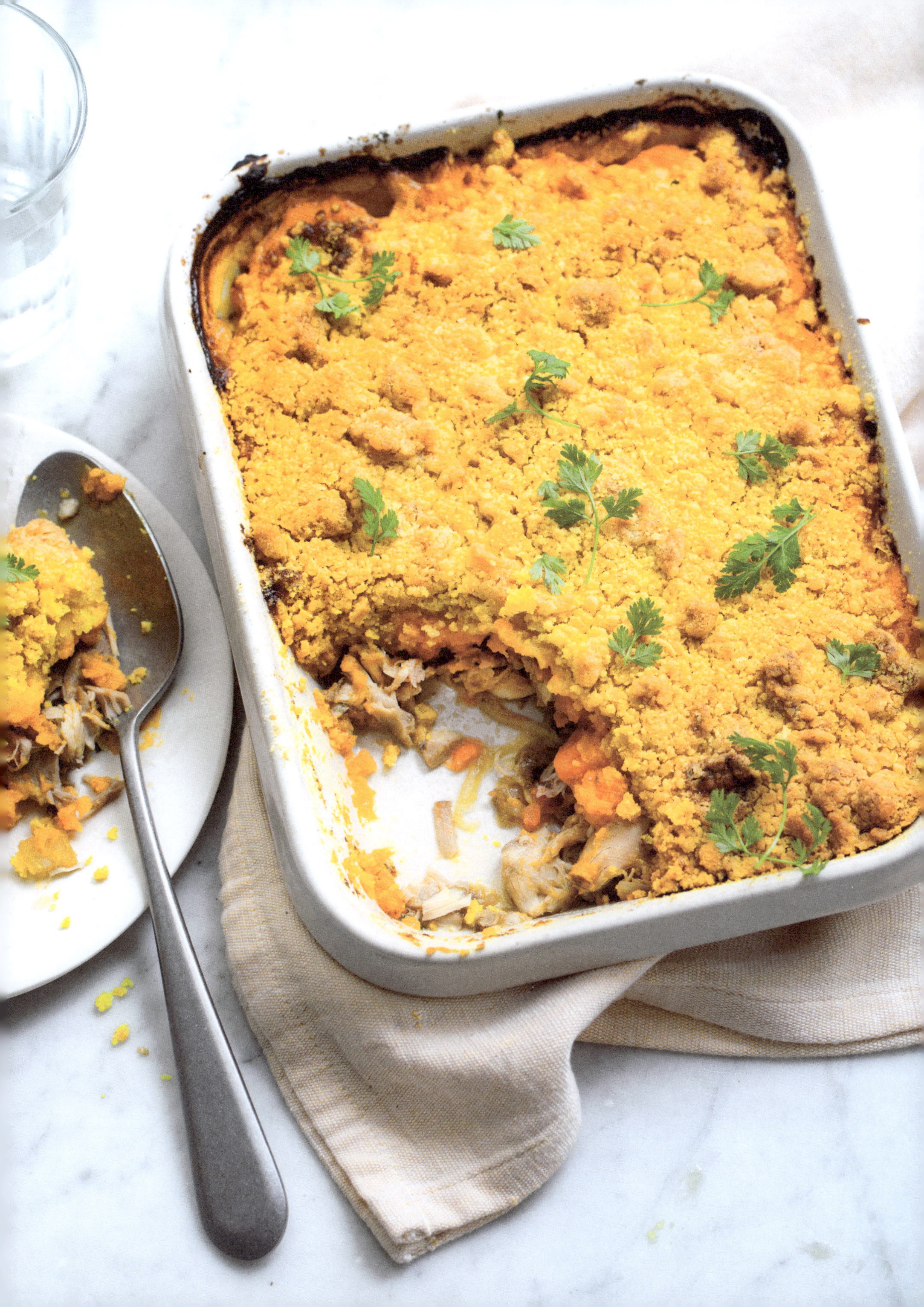

As a supplement

To boost production

Citrus Osso Buco

SERVES **2** • PREPARATION TIME: **15 MINUTES**
COOKING TIME: **2 HOURS 10 MINUTES**

2 veal shanks
50 g (2 oz) plain flour
2 tablespoons olive oil
½ onion, finely chopped
2 garlic cloves, finely chopped
1 carrot, peeled and cut into large chunks
2 celery sticks, cut into large chunks
100 ml (3½ fl oz) red wine
400g (13 oz) can of crushed tomatoes
500 ml French-style 'Pot-au-Feu' Broth (see page 17)
salt and pepper

FOR THE GREMOLATA

finely chopped zest of 1 lemon
finely chopped zest of 1 orange
1 bunch of parsley, finely chopped

1. Dip the shanks into the flour and tap to remove the excess.
2. Heat the oil in a casserole dish. When hot, brown the shanks on both sides until golden brown, then remove and set aside.
3. Sauté the vegetables in the same oil for 3 minutes.
4. Place the meat back in the dish, pour in the wine and add the crushed tomatoes and stock. Season with salt and pepper. Cover and cook for at least 1½ hours over a medium heat.
5. To make the gremolata, mix the citrus zests with the chopped parsley.
6. Add the gremolata to the casserole dish and cook for a further 30 minutes.

Tip

Serve with a creamy polenta.

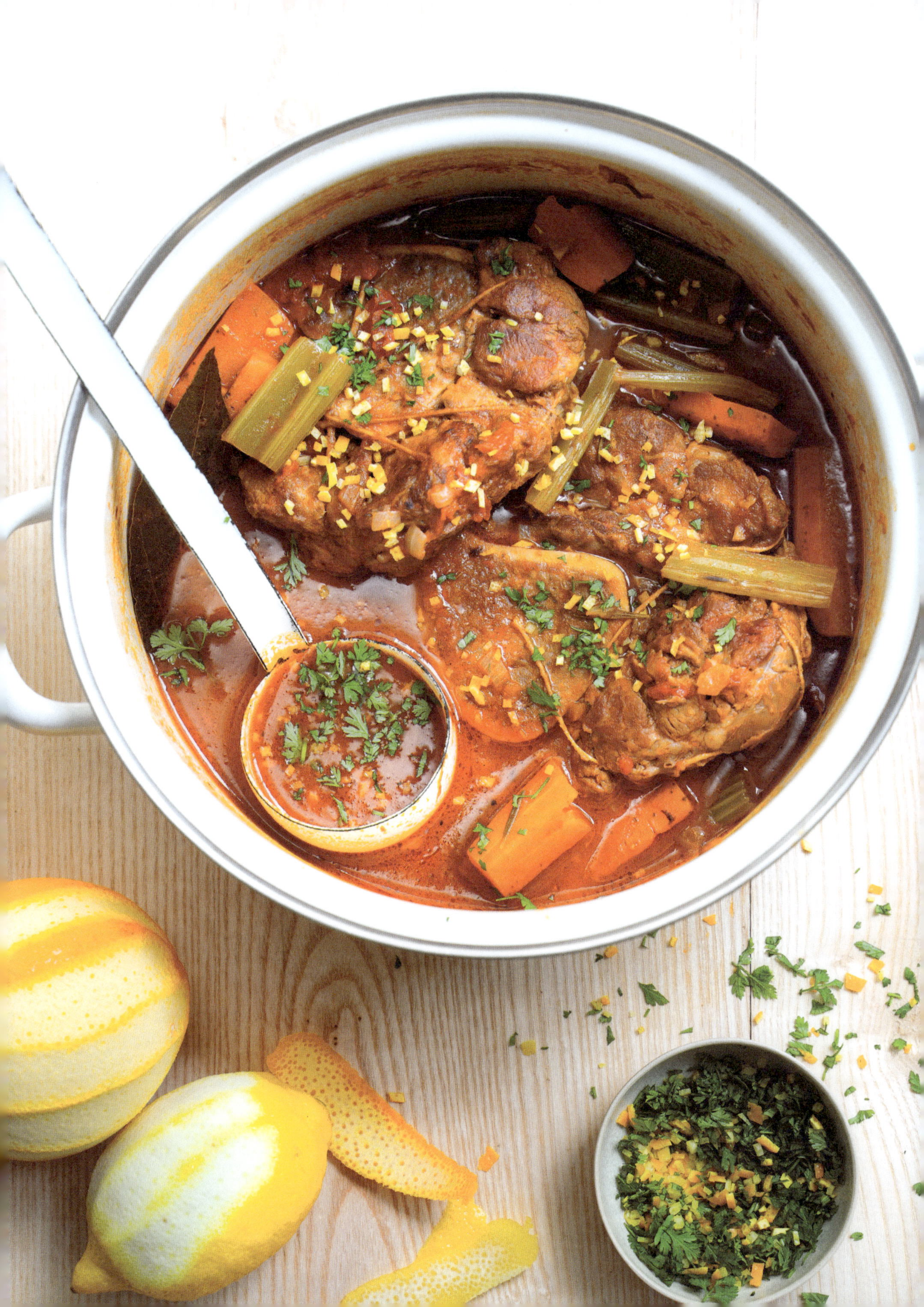

As a supplement

To boost production

Chicken, Carrot and Grilled Lemon Tagine

SERVES **2** • PREPARATION TIME: **20 MINUTES** • COOKING TIME: **50 MINUTES**

½ lemon
1 tablespoon olive oil
2 skin-on, bone-in chicken thighs
4 carrots, peeled and sliced on the diagonal
1 onion, cut into wedges
1 garlic clove, peeled and halved
½ teaspoon ground turmeric
½ teaspoon ras el hanout
½ teaspoon ground cumin
1 cinnamon stick
500 ml (17 fl oz) Chicken Stock (see page 16)
2 tablespoons cranberries
4 ready-to-eat dried apricots
pinch of coarse salt
100 g (3½ oz) drained canned chickpeas

1. Char the lemon half in a dry casserole dish for 3 minutes until blackened, then remove and set aside.
2. Add the oil to the dish and sauté the chicken thighs for 5 minutes, starting skin-side down. Turn them over and continue to cook for 1–2 minutes before removing from the pan.
3. Sauté the carrots, onion and garlic for 2 minutes until they are evenly coloured, then reduce the heat and add the spices. Pour in the stock and deglaze the dish, scraping the bottom with a spatula.
4. Put the meat back in the casserole dish along with the cranberries, apricots, grilled lemon and a pinch of coarse salt. Cover and cook for 25 minutes.
5. Add the chickpeas and remove the lid. Reduce for a final 10 minutes.

Tip

Serve with 200 g (7 oz) couscous or cooked bulgur wheat mixed with 1 tablespoon olive oil.

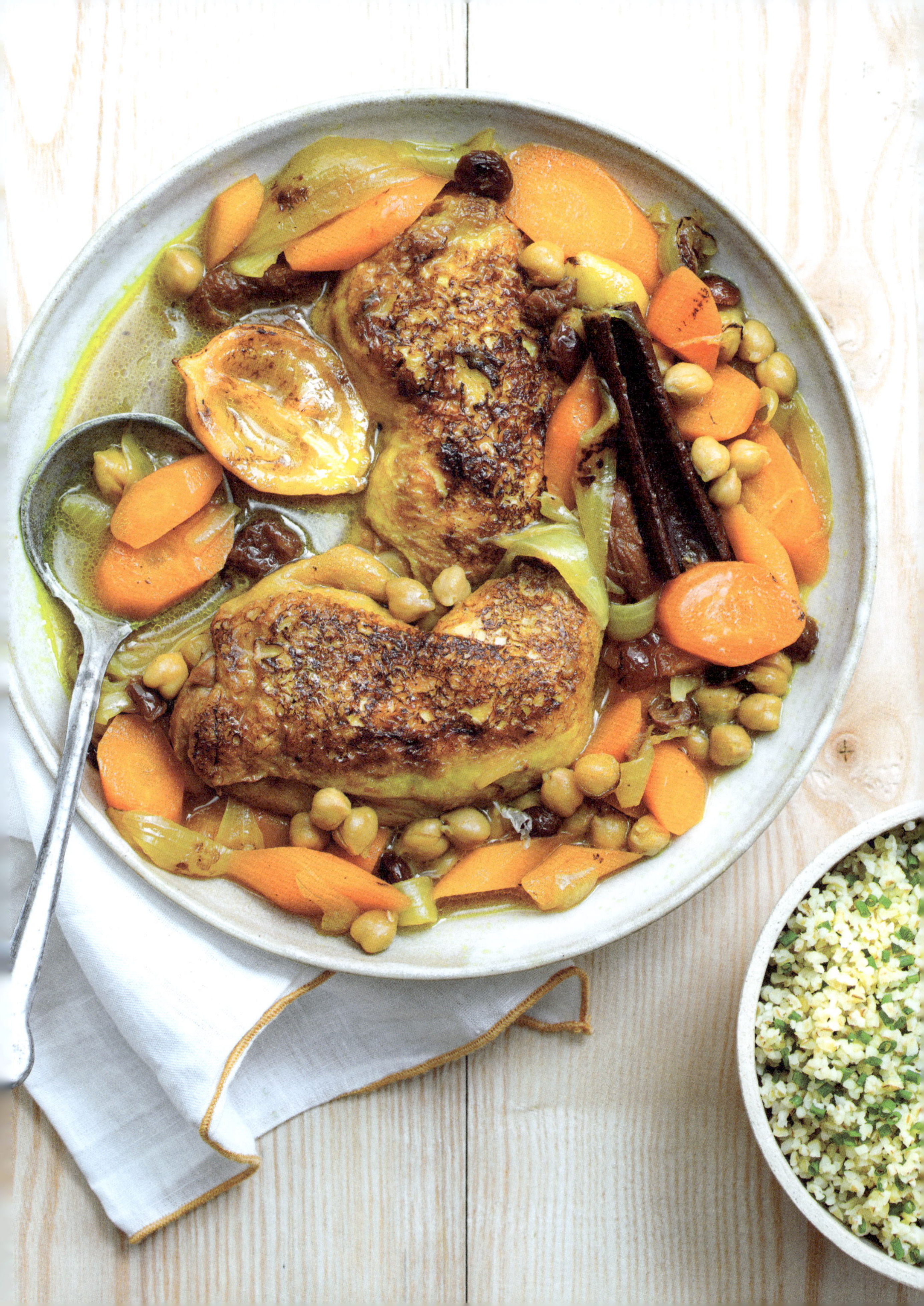

Spicy Braised Beef Noodle Soup

SERVES **2** • PREPARATION TIME: **10 MINUTES** • COOKING TIME: **30 MINUTES**

1 tablespoon oil
½ onion, finely chopped
3 garlic cloves, finely chopped
3 cm (1 inch) fresh root ginger, peeled and finely chopped
3 tablespoons concentrated tomato paste
2 tablespoons chilli paste (optional)
1 tablespoon sugar
8 tablespoons soy sauce
800 ml (28 fl oz) beef Phô Broth (see page 18)
250 g (8 oz) shredded beef from the Phô Broth (see page 18)
½ small Chinese cabbage, halved
50 g (2 oz) thick wheat noodles
6 coriander sprigs
coarse salt

1. Heat the oil in a casserole dish. When hot, sauté the onion, garlic and ginger for 2 minutes over a medium heat, then add the tomato paste and chilli paste, if desired, and cook for a further 2 minutes.
2. Add the sugar, soy sauce, stock and meat. Cover and simmer for 25 minutes.
3. Meanwhile, cook the Chinese cabbage in salted boiling water for 5 minutes.
4. Cook the noodles according to the packet instructions.
5. Divide the noodles and Chinese cabbage between 2 bowls. Pour in the soup and garnish with coriander.

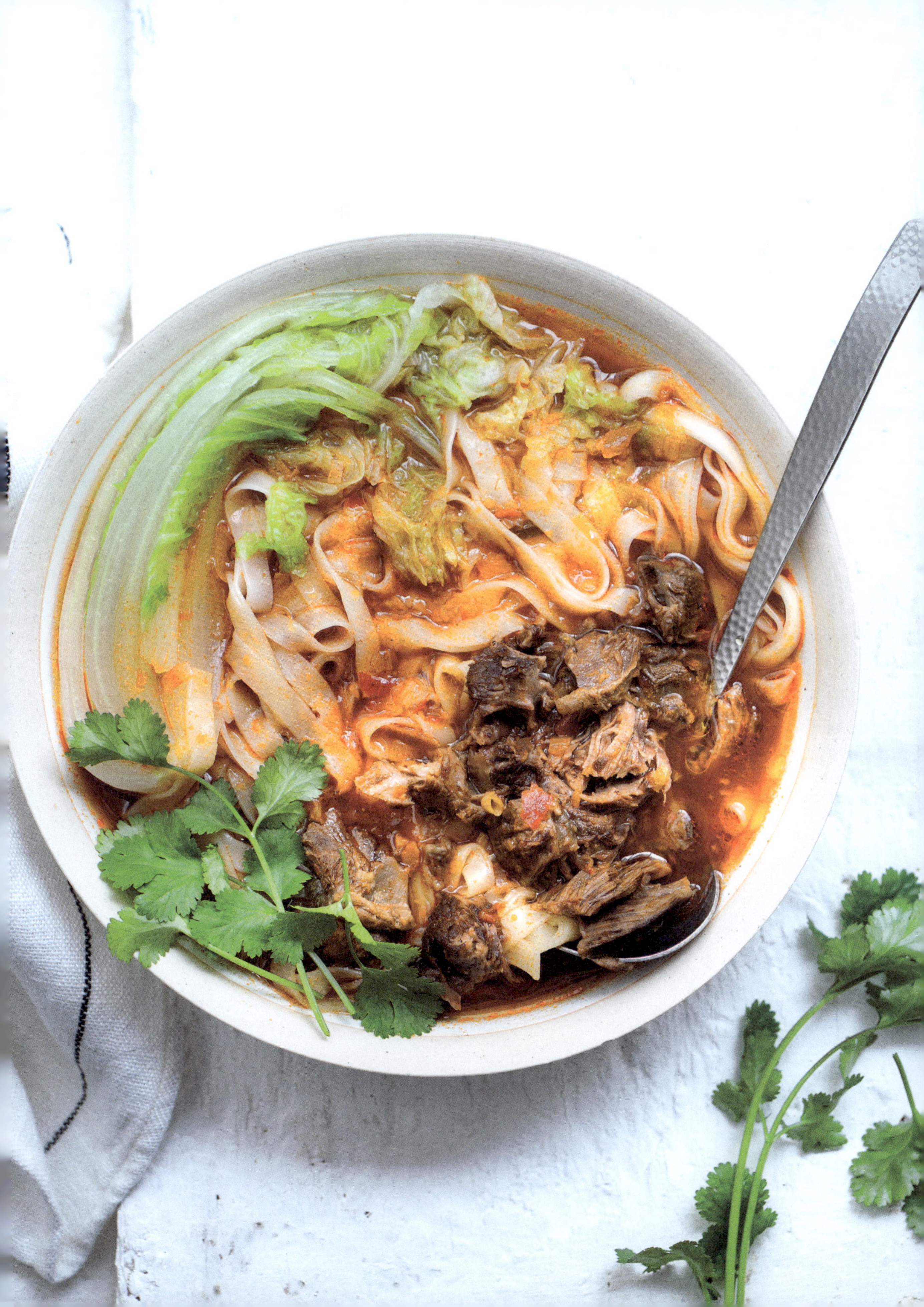

COLLAGEN THERAPY • WINTER

Immunity, vitality and digestion

Winter is the season when the immune system needs extra support. This treatment focuses on protecting the immune system, cell renewal and stimulating collagen production to combat skin dryness and fatigue.

AIM

To stimulate the immune system, prevent collagen degradation and maintain energy levels.

As a supplement

KEY FOODS

The following foods contain bioactive collagen and essential amino acids for the reconstruction of connective tissues.

Fish, including the skin and bones
(salmon, sardines, mackerel) (rich in anti-inflammatory Type I collagen and Omega-3)

Bone broth
(beef, chicken, fish) (rich in Types I and II collagen, ideal for joints)

Egg white
(rich in proline, a precursor to collagen)

Pork rind
(baked, jellied, in homemade pâté)

Natural gelatine and collagen powder

To boost production

KEY NUTRIENTS

To stimulate collagen production naturally, some essential cofactors are required.

- **Vitamin C** (citrus fruit, red berries, peppers, parsley and broccoli)
- **Zinc and copper** (oysters, seeds, dark chocolate, cashew nuts, sunflower seeds, lean red meat)
- **Silica** (oats, cucumber, carrots, nuts, seeds)
- **Omega-3 fatty acids** (oily fish, avocado, flaxseed)
- **Antioxidants** (green tea, berries, raw cacao, carrots, turmeric)

	DAY 1	DAY 2
BREAKFAST	Spirulina Latte • see page 29 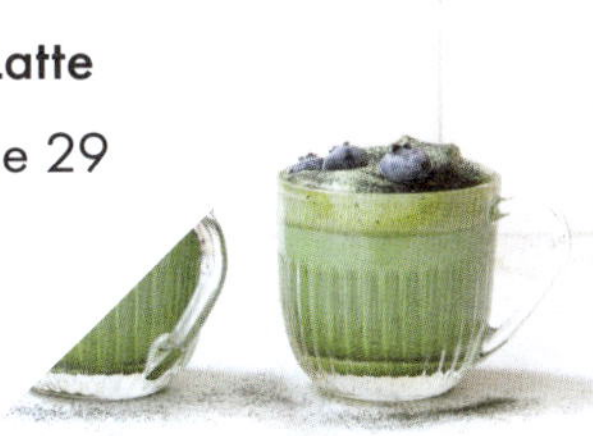	Bowl of kefir, Brazil nuts, goji berries and fresh fruit
LUNCH	Thai-style Prawn Broth • see page 21 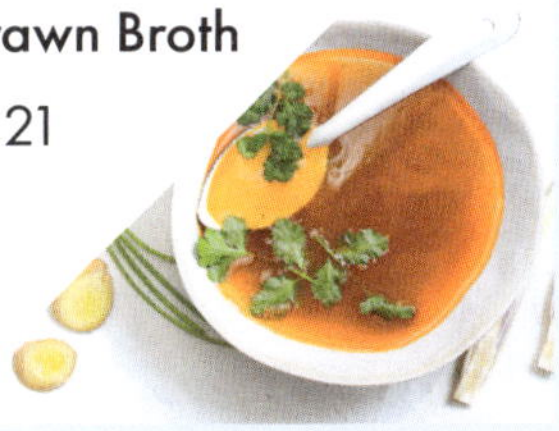	Shredded Chicken Congee • see page 38 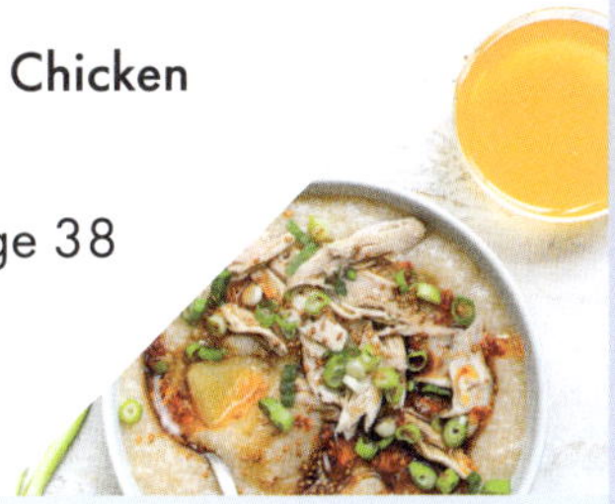
SNACK	Baked pineapple and grated coconut	Chocolate Fondant Squares • see page 120 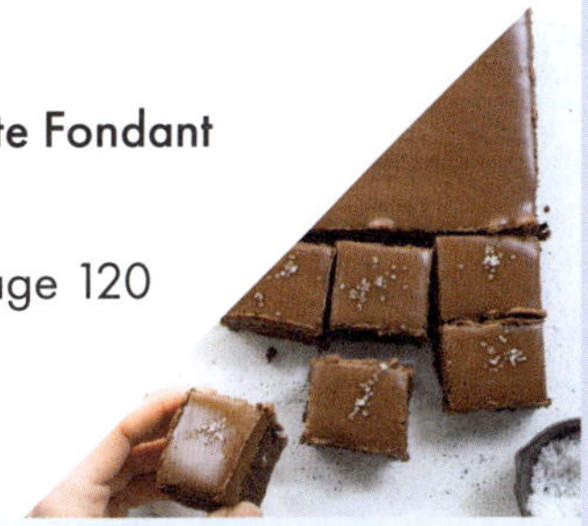
DINNER	Citrus Osso Buco • see page 130 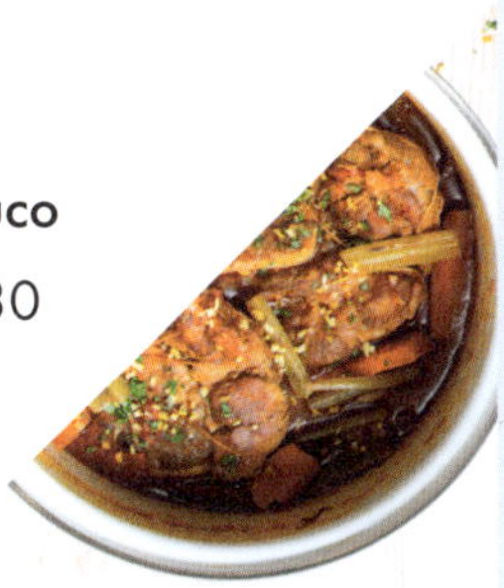	Mackerel fillet, broccoli purée and lemon juice

Crab Cakes, Avocado and Mango Salad

SERVES **2** • PREPARATION TIME: **25 MINUTES** • COOKING TIME: **12 MINUTES**

FOR THE AVOCADO AND MANGO SALAD

150 g (5 oz) frozen broad beans (or edamame)
1 avocado, peeled, pitted and diced
½ mango (about 160 g/5½ oz), diced
3 basil or mint sprigs, roughly chopped
juice of 1 lime
1 teaspoon nuoc-mâm (Vietnamese dipping sauce)
1 tablespoon soy sauce
1 tablespoon sesame oil

FOR THE CRAB CAKES

175 g (6 oz) crab meat
10 g (½ oz) fresh root ginger, peeled and grated
1 egg yolk
1 tablespoon Sriracha sauce
50 g (2 oz) mayonnaise
zest of 1 lime
½ red onion, finely chopped
40 g (1½ oz) breadcrumbs
6 chives, chopped
salt and pepper
3 tablespoons sunflower oil

1. To prepare the avocado and mango salad, cook the broad beans (or edamame) for 5 minutes in a small saucepan of boiling water. Drain and tip into a bowl of cold water to halt the cooking process.
2. Mix the drained beans with the remaining salad ingredients and leave to rest in the refrigerator.
3. In a large bowl, mix the crab, ginger, egg yolk, Sriracha, mayo, lime zest, red onion, breadcrumbs and chives. Season with salt and pepper, then shape the mixture into small, flat patties.
4. Heat the oil in a frying pan over a high heat. Add the crab cakes and cook for about 3 minutes on each side.
5. Serve the crab cakes with the salad.

Tip

Why not make your own mayo? Whisk 1 egg yolk at room temperature with 1 teaspoon of Dijon mustard. Gradually incorporate 100 ml (3½ fl oz) of sunflower oil by slowly pouring it in a thin, steady stream, whisking all the time to ensure the mayonnaise is properly emulsified. Season with salt and pepper.

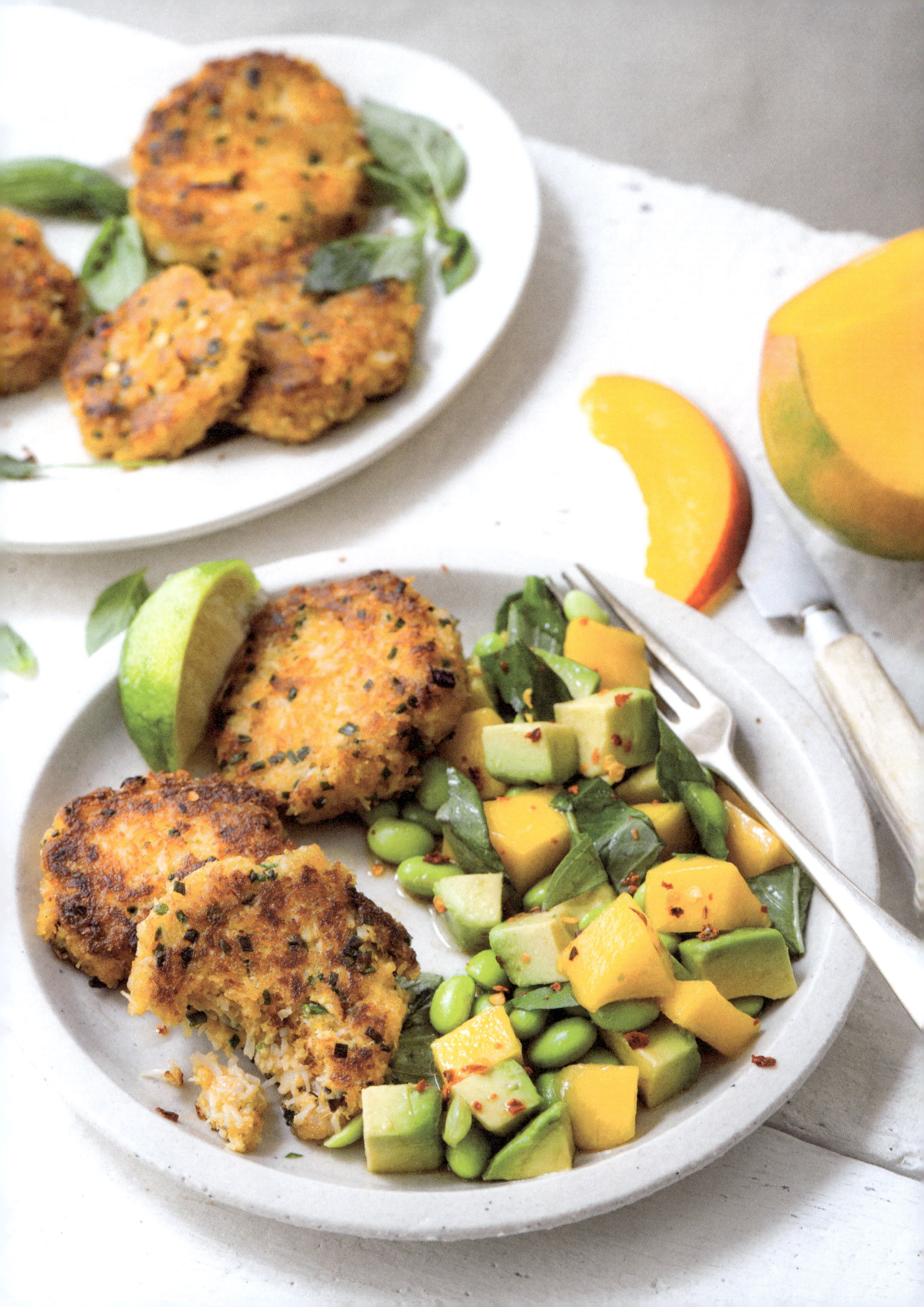

To boost production

Oysters in Watercress Jelly

SERVES **2** • PREPARATION TIME: **20 MINUTES** • COOKING TIME: **5 MINUTES**
RESTING TIME **1½ HOURS**

12 oysters
½ bunch of watercress
3 gelatine leaves
200 ml (7 fl oz) Fish Stock (see page 20)
coarse salt, to serve
handful of watercress sprouts or sprouted seeds, to garnish

FOR THE TOMATO SALSA

1 green tomato, deseeded and diced
1 yellow tomato, deseeded and diced
½ shallot, finely chopped
2 tablespoons good-quality olive oil
salt and pepper

1. Open the oysters and reserve their liquid by straining it through a fine sieve. Detach the oysters from the shells and set aside in the refrigerator. Rinse the hollow parts of the shells and leave to dry.
2. Wash the watercress, cut the stems and keep only the leaves. Drop the leaves into a saucepan of salted boiling water and cook for 5 minutes. Drain, then transfer the leaves to a bowl of cold water to fix the colour. Drain and reserve some watercress leaves for the salad. Blend the rest together to a smooth, vibrant green purée.
3. Rehydrate the gelatine in a bowl of cold water.
4. Heat the Fish Stock in a small saucepan, then dissolve the drained gelatine in it. Leave to cool, then combine with the watercress purée.
5. Place the washed shells on a bed of coarse salt to keep them level. Pour in the watercress jelly and place in the refrigerator for 1½ hours.
6. To make the salsa: mix the tomatoes, shallot and oil with the reserved, chopped watercress leaves. Season with salt and pepper.
7. Place the oysters on the set jelly and garnish with the salsa and a few sprouts.

Tip

You can use the leftover watercress stems in the soup on page 102.

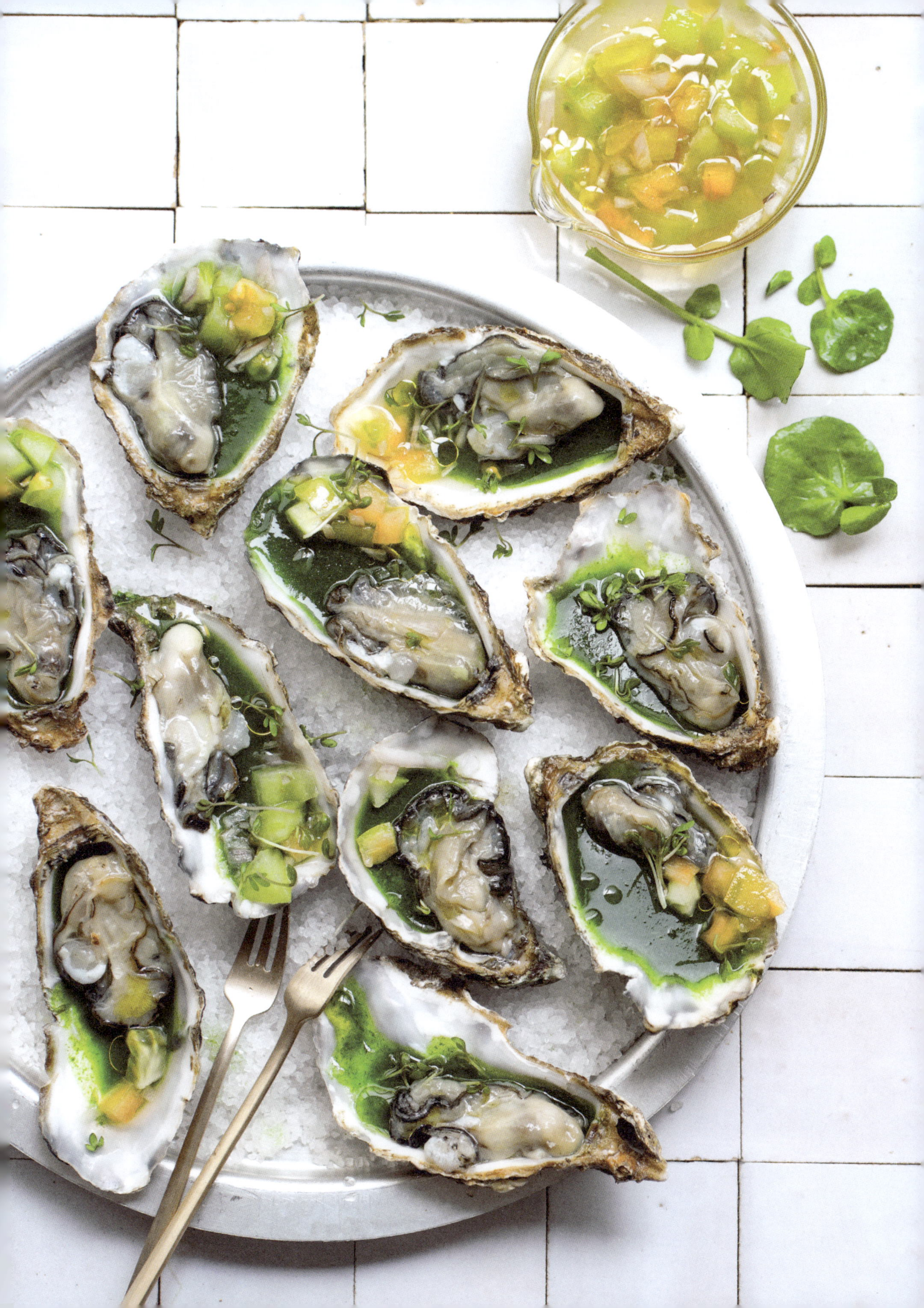

To **boost** production

Herring and Lentil Salad

SERVES **2** • PREPARATION TIME: **15 MINUTES** • COOKING TIME: **25 MINUTES**
RESTING TIME: **1½ HOURS**

100 g (3½ oz) green lentils
2 sweet herring fillets, cut into bite-sized pieces
1 cooked red beetroot, diced
60 g (2¼ oz) red cabbage, thinly sliced
5 rainbow radishes, quartered
¼ bunch of watercress (leaves only)
4 tarragon sprigs (or use dill), finely chopped

FOR THE QUICK-PICKLED RED ONION

½ red onion, peeled and chopped into thin wedges
20 g (¾ oz) sugar
40 ml (1½ fl oz) white vinegar
80 ml (3 fl oz) water

FOR THE VINAIGRETTE

1 teaspoon horseradish
3 tablespoons cider vinegar
4 tablespoons flaxseed or rapeseed oil
salt and pepper

1. To make the quick pickle, place the red onion wedges in a glass jar. Mix the sugar, vinegar and water in a small saucepan and bring to the boil. As soon as the sugar has dissolved, pour the hot liquid over the onion. Seal, cool and place in the refrigerator for at least 1½ hours.
2. Cook the lentils in a large pan of unsalted boiling water for 20–25 minutes, according to the packet instructions.
3. Make the vinaigrette by mixing all the ingredients together in a large bowl.
4. Add the still warm, drained lentils to the bowl of vinaigrette, combine well and leave to cool completely.
5. Incorporate the rest of the salad ingredients with the lentils, including the drained pickled red onion, before serving.

Tip

Avoid adding salt to the lentil cooking water, as this would prolong the cooking time. By mixing the warm lentils with the vinaigrette, the vinaigrette will be better absorbed and your salad will be tastier.

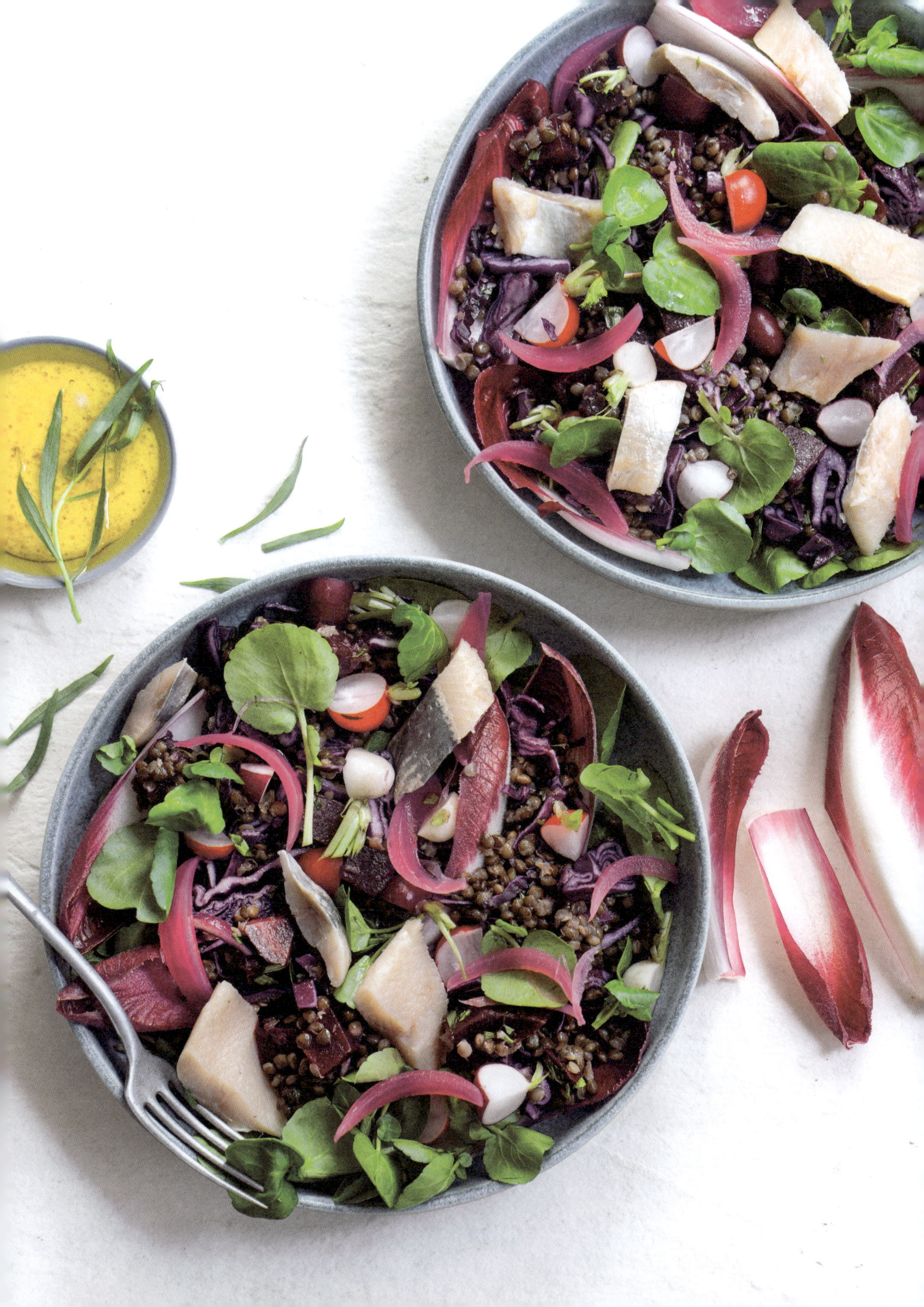

Miso, Mushroom and Tofu Soup

SERVES **2** • PREPARATION TIME: **10 MINUTES** • COOKING TIME: **15 MINUTES**

FOR THE BROTH

400 ml (14 fl oz) Vegetarian Dashi (see page 22)
30 g (1 ¼ oz) red miso
5 g (¼ oz) fresh root ginger, peeled and finely chopped
300 ml (½ pint) Vegetable Stock (see page 23)
4 button mushrooms (or any other medium-sized mushroom), sliced
50 g (2 oz) small mushrooms (such as shimeji or small button mushrooms)
1 tablespoon wakame (dried seaweed) (optional)
1 leek top (green part), washed and julienned
160 g (5½ oz) buckwheat soba noodles

FOR THE MARINATED TOFU

100 g (3 ½ oz) silken tofu, cut into large cubes
2 tablespoons soy sauce
1 tablespoon sesame oil

1. Pour the Dashi into a saucepan and gently heat with the miso and ginger for about 15 minutes, with the lid on, making sure it does not boil.
2. Pour the vegetable stock into another saucepan, add the mushrooms, seaweed and leek top, bring to the boil and cook for 15 minutes over a medium heat.
3. Meanwhile, mix the diced tofu with the soy sauce and sesame oil.
4. Cook the soba noodles in a large saucepan of boiling water according to the packet instructions.
5. Divide the noodles between 2 bowls, then divide the broths between them. Add the marinated tofu and serve.

Tip

For a more protein-rich version, add 2 fillets of sea bass or sea bream that have already been poached in the Dashi.

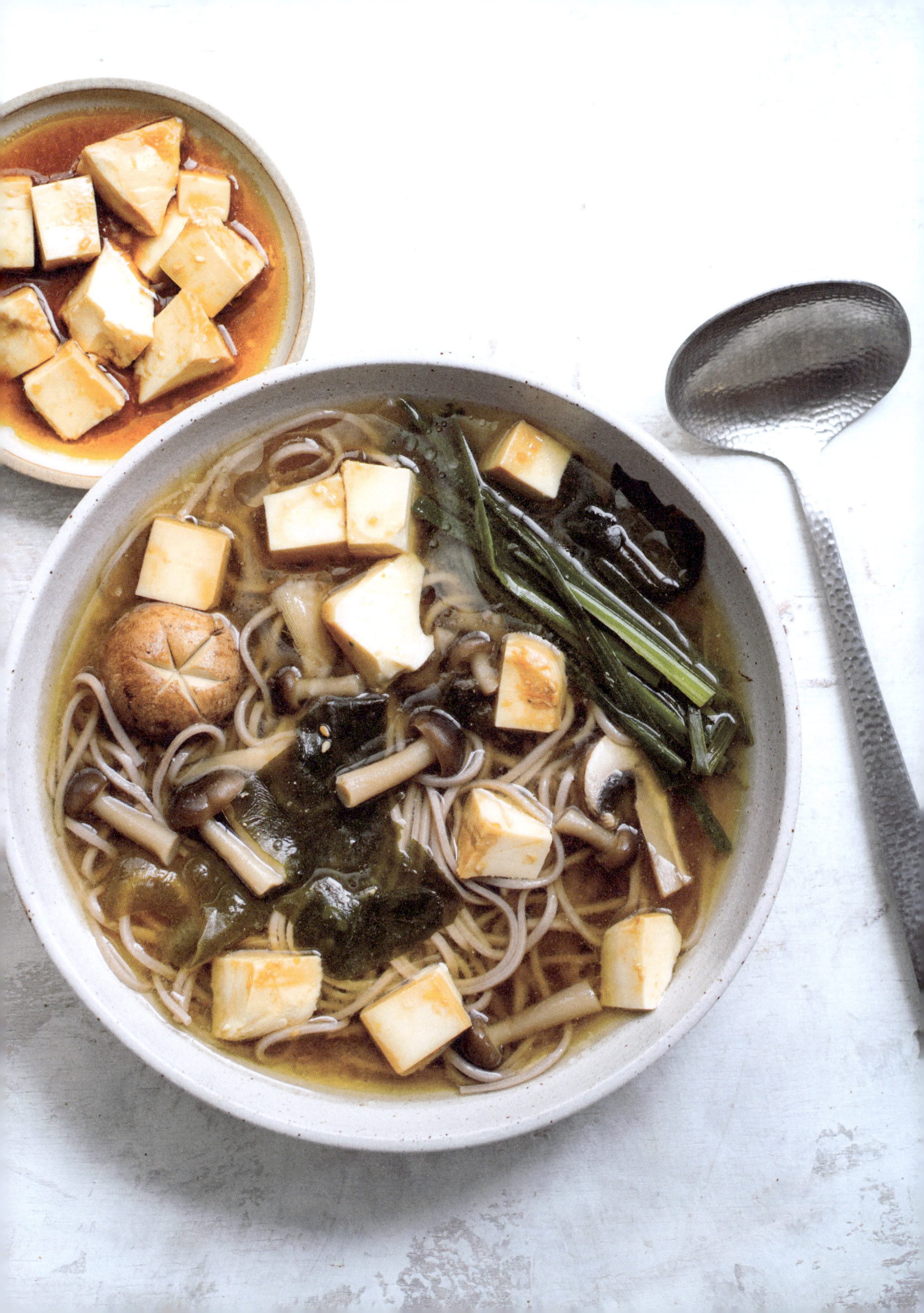

To **boost** production

Mapo Tofu

SERVES **2** • PREPARATION TIME: **15 MINUTES** • COOKING TIME: **35 MINUTES**
RESTING TIME: **5 MINUTES**

- 150 g (5 oz) brown rice
- 400 g (13 oz) soft tofu, cut into large cubes
- ½ teaspoon fine salt
- 2 tablespoons neutral oil (such as sunflower)
- 2 garlic cloves, finely chopped
- 10 g (½ oz) fresh root ginger, peeled and finely chopped
- 1 tablespoon Sichuan pepper
- 2 tablespoons concentrated tomato paste
- 400 ml (14 fl oz) Vegetable Stock (see page 23)
- 100 g (3½ oz) drained canned white, kidney or black beans
- 1 tablespoon cornflour
- 2 spring onions, finely chopped

1. Cook the brown rice according to the packet instructions.
2. Place the tofu in a bowl, cover with very hot water and add the salt. Leave to rest for 5 minutes, then carefully drain.
3. Heat the oil in a saucepan. When hot, sauté the garlic and ginger for 1 minute, then add the Sichuan pepper and tomato paste. Stir for 1 minute.
4. Add the Vegetable Stock, beans and tofu to the pan and simmer for about 15 minutes over a medium heat, gently stirring.
5. Remove about 100 ml (3½ fl oz) of the cooking liquid and pour into a small bowl. Add the cornflour and mix until thoroughly combined.
6. Gradually incorporate the cornflour mixture back into the saucepan, stirring until the sauce has thickened. Sprinkle with the spring onions and serve with the cooked rice.

Tip

For a more traditional stew, add 2 tablespoons chilli sauce of your choice at the beginning of the cooking.

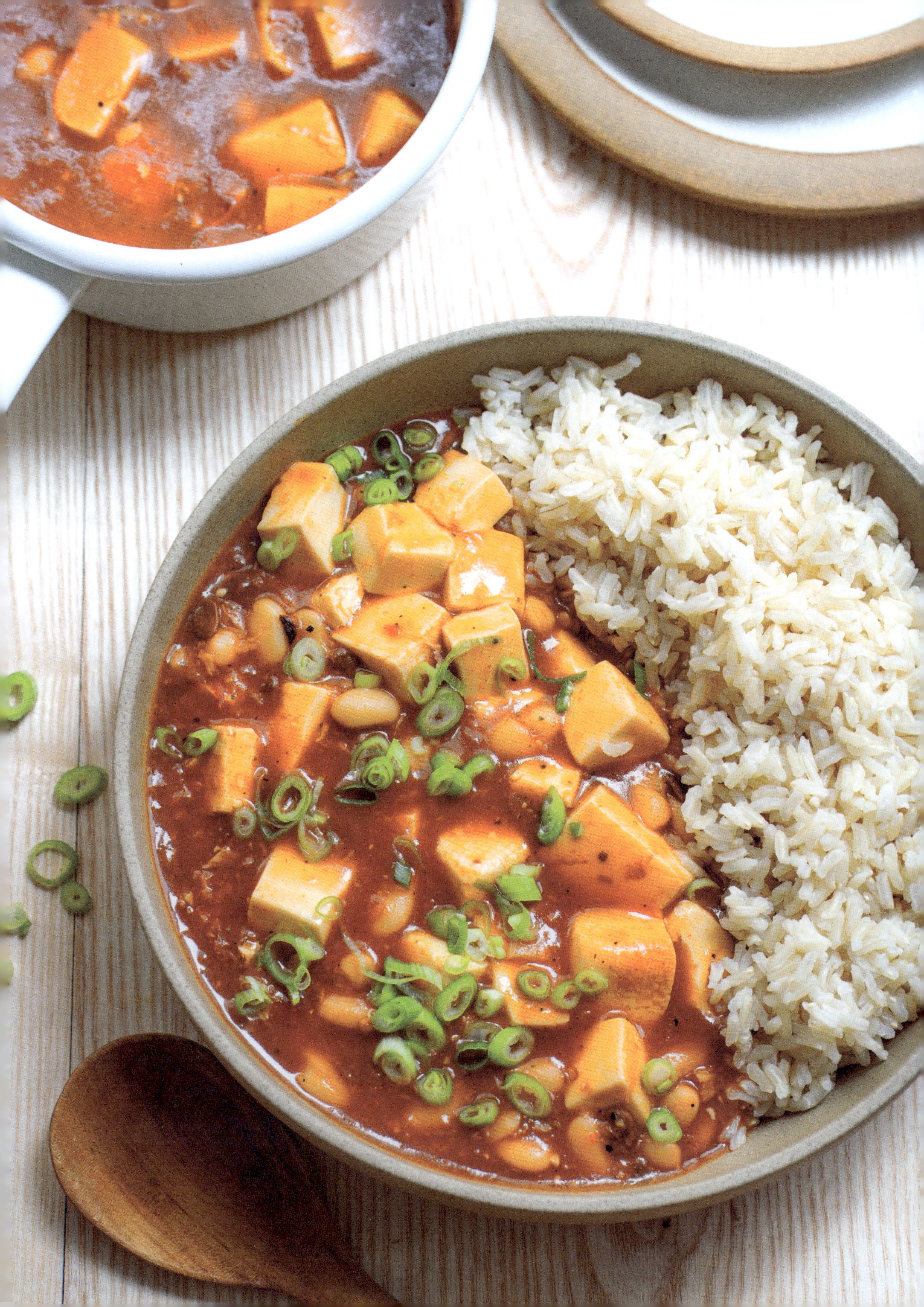

Pearl Barley Minestrone with Squash

As a supplement

To boost production

SERVES **2** • PREPARATION TIME: **15 MINUTES** • COOKING TIME: **45 MINUTES**

1 tablespoon olive oil
1 onion, finely chopped
1 carrot, peeled and finely diced
1 celery stick, strings removed, finely sliced
50 g (2 oz) pancetta, diced
250 g (8 oz) squash, peeled and diced
75 g (3 oz) pearl barley
1 small rosemary sprig
1 bay leaf
750 ml (1 ¼ pints) Vegetable Stock (see page 23) or stock of your choice
100 g (3 ½ oz) drained canned white beans
freshly ground pepper

1. Heat the oil in a saucepan over a medium heat. When hot, sauté the onion, carrot, celery and pancetta for 5 minutes.
2. Add the squash, pearl barley, rosemary sprig and bay leaf. Season with pepper, cover with the Vegetable Stock and simmer for 35 minutes, with the lid on.
3. Add the white beans and continue to cook for a final 5 minutes.

Tip

To add more flavour to your minestrone, you can add a piece of Parmesan rind during the cooking.

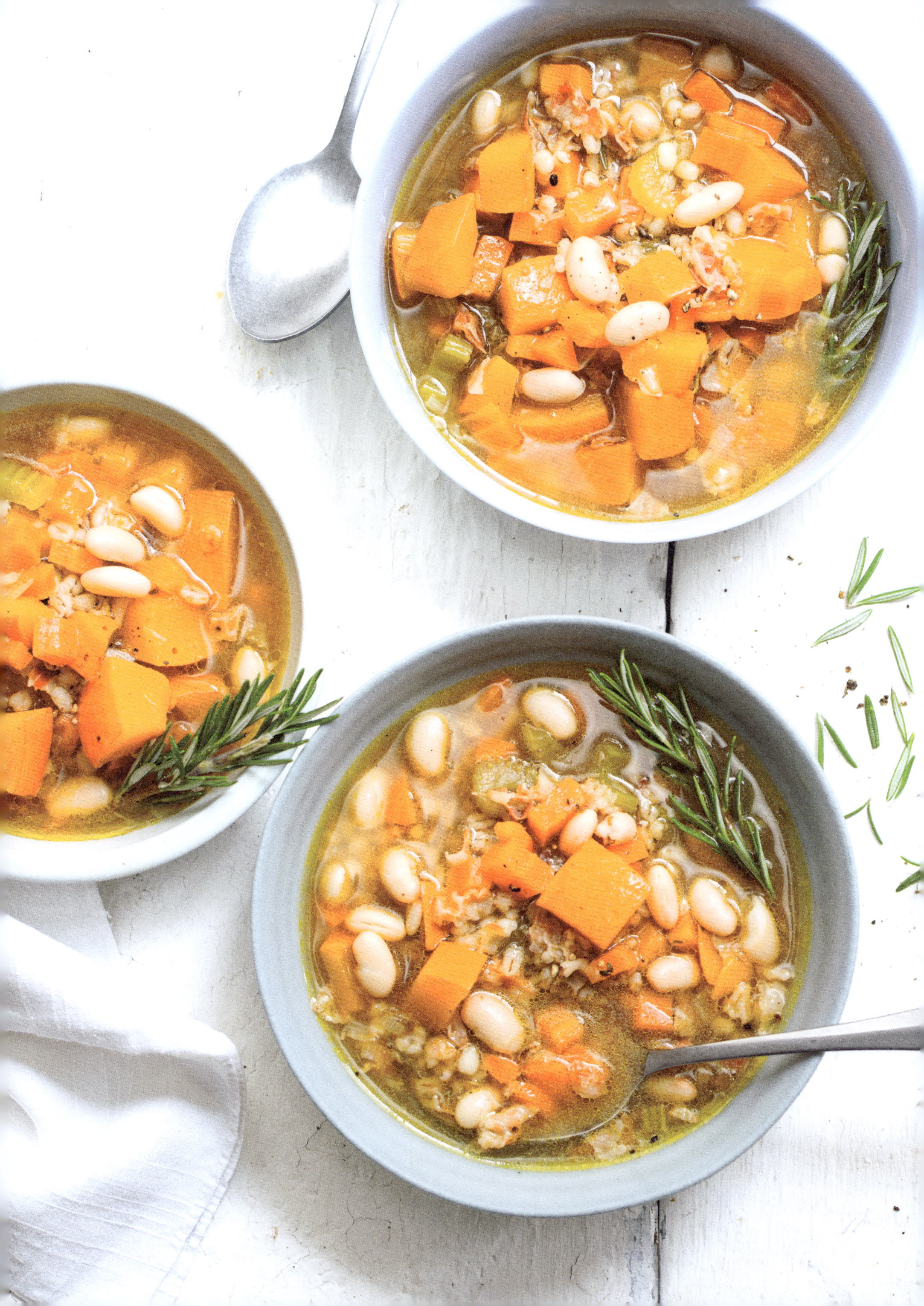

As a supplement

To boost production

Coconut and Mango Flan

SERVES **3** • PREPARATION TIME: **15 MINUTES** • COOKING TIME: **5 MINUTES**
RESTING TIME: **1 HOUR 40 MINUTES**

6 g (¼ oz) powdered gelatine
80 ml (3 fl oz) cold water
230 g (7½ oz) mango, peeled and roughly chopped
120 ml (4 fl oz) coconut milk
15 g (½ oz) powdered milk
12 g (½ oz) cane sugar
¼ teaspoon Chinese 5-Spice
pinch of sea salt flakes

TO DECORATE

2 tablespoons coconut cream
50 g (2 oz) mango, peeled and diced
a few mint sprigs
a few coconut flakes

1. Rehydrate the gelatine in the measured cold water. Leave to soak for about 10 minutes.
2. Place the mango in a blender and blitz to a purée.
3. Combine the coconut milk, powdered milk, sugar, spices and salt in a saucepan and heat until the sugar has dissolved. Remove from the heat, and incorporate the gelatine until dissolved, then add the mango purée.
4. Divide the mango mixture among serving dishes, decorate each one with a dash of coconut cream and place in the refrigerator for at least 1½ hours.
5. When ready to serve, decorate with mint leaves, a few pieces of fresh mango, coconut flakes and another dash of coconut cream, if desired.

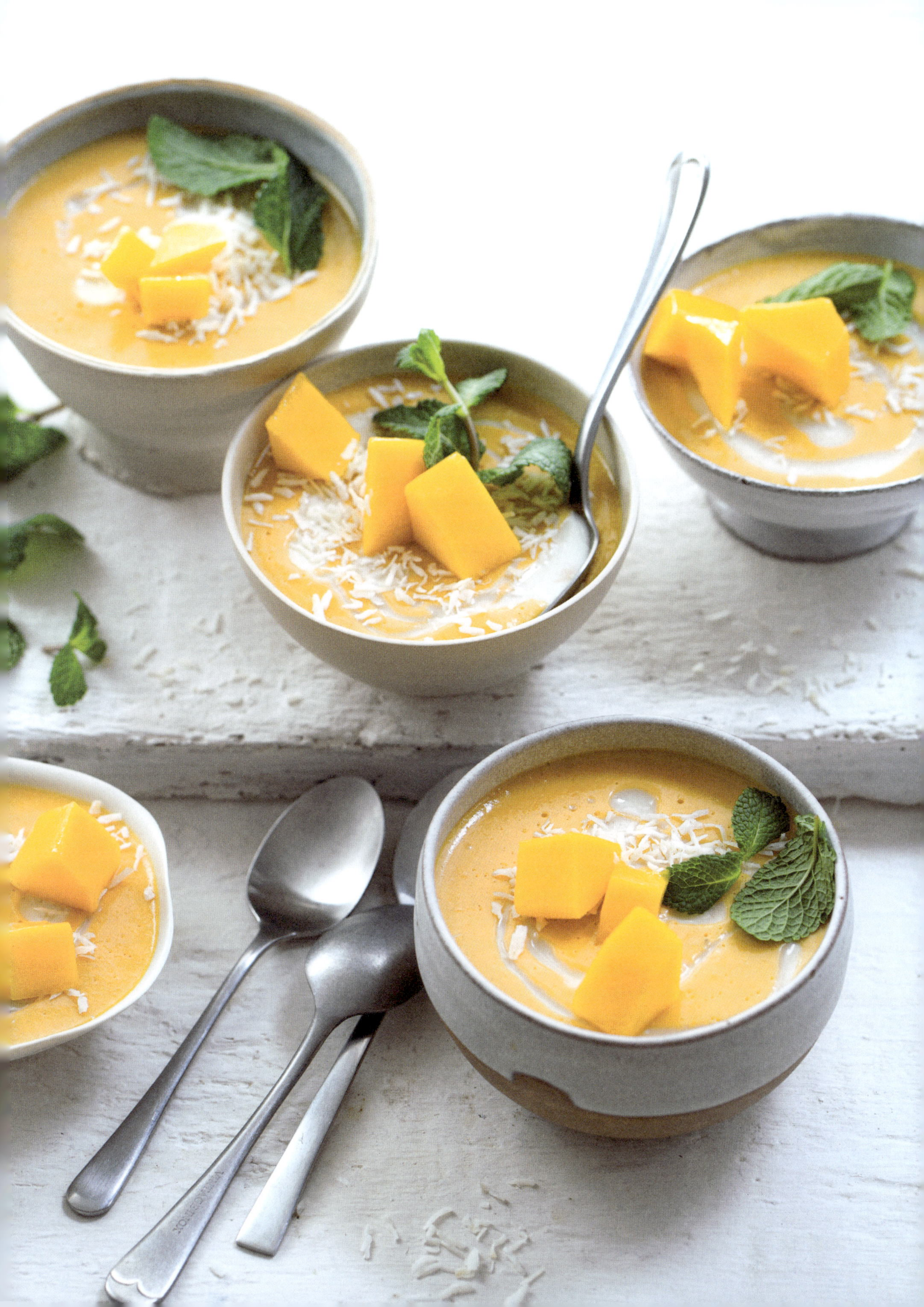

Appendices

Table of recipes

Index

First published in Great Britain in 2026 by Hamlyn,
an imprint of Octopus Publishing Group Ltd,
Carmelite House, 50 Victoria Embankment,
London, EC4Y 0DZ
www.octopusbooks.co.uk

An Hachette UK Company
www.hachette.co.uk

The authorized representative in the EEA is
Hachette Ireland, 8 Castlecourt Centre, Dublin 15,
D15 XTP3, Ireland
(email: info@hbgi.ie)

Originally published in France as *Mes Recettes Collagène*
by Marabout, 58, rue Jean-Bleuzen, CS 70007, 92178
Vanves Cedex. France
contact@marabout.fr

Copyright for original French edition
© Hachette Livre (Marabout) 2025

Copyright for this English edition
© Octopus Publishing Group Ltd 2026

Distributed in the US by Hachette Book Group,
1290 Avenue of the Americas, 4th and 5th Floors,
New York, NY 10104

Distributed in Canada by Canadian Manda Group,
664 Annette St., Toronto, Ontario, Canada M6S 2C8

All rights reserved. No part of this work may be reproduced or utilized in any form or by any means, electronic or mechanical, including photocopying, recording or by any information storage and retrieval system, without the prior written permission of the publisher.

Séverine Augé and Elodie Colombel assert the moral right to be identified as the authors of this work.

ISBN 978-0-600-64037-0
eISBN 978-0-600-64045-5

A CIP catalogue record for this book is available from the British Library.

Printed and bound in China.

10 9 8 7 6 5 4 3 2 1

For Hamlyn:
Publisher: Kate Fox
Assistant Editor: Alice Gawthrop
Art Director: Jaz Bahra
Editor: Rosie Hilton
Translation from the French: First Editions Translations
Production Manager: Caroline Alberti
Photography: Fabrice Besse
Food styling: Séverine Augé

For Marabout:
Editing: Céline de Quéral
Page layout and design: Claire Fauvain